STAYING YOUNG

Staying Young

Lifestyle Changes for Turning Back the Clock

Dr. Courtney A. Mote

ISBN: 1530239567
ISBN 13: 9781530239566

DEDICATION

To my fabulous mother and father, who have always supported me 100 percent, regardless of how reckless and obsessive-compulsive I have been all my life.

To my superb medical staff at Spectrum Healthcare, who have yet to fire me from the clinic I own.

To those who choose to be like Peter Pan and never grow old—may you join me in this journey.

Introduction

You've probably heard the saying, "You're only as young as you feel." No truer words have ever been spoken. When it comes to feeling youthful now and for many years to come, you cannot focus on one aspect of healthy living and avoid all others. You must look to your diet, fitness, mental and emotional well-being, and the environment you place yourself in when looking to improve your overall health and vitality.

Looking and feeling young are greatly influenced by one's lifestyle choices. If you want to feel young and healthy, you can. Whatever your age, you can slow the aging process. You can look and feel younger than you do today. Whether you are in your twenties and just want to keep that vibrant feeling of youth, or eighty years of age and looking for ways to turn back the clock, this book is for you.

You are obviously interested in the idea of anti-aging, otherwise, you wouldn't have picked up this book. You have already taken the first step. As with anything you research and educate yourself on, you must act on what you learn. So remember to envision yourself with a slightly different lifestyle than the one you currently have—one that focuses on your body, mind, and spirit.

In this book, we'll cover a wide range of things pertaining to looking and feeling younger. We will go over the nutrition, the physical activity, the mind-set, and the skin treatments and therapies that, when put together (like the pieces of a puzzle), will greatly improve your well-being. Just by focusing on a couple different aspects addressed in this book, you will enjoy stellar results. Remember, you don't have to change everything at once. You can slowly add small alterations into your lifestyle at whatever speed you feel is best for you.

How You Should Read This Book

If you are starving for information that will guide and motivate you toward better health, you should carefully consider the information in this book. Simply reading a book on healthy living or anti-aging will not magically result in your becoming healthier and younger-looking without applying the information you've read. Thus, I recommend you read this book by focusing on one chapter at a time. With each chapter, read it somewhat quickly. Then go back and read said chapter again but more slowly this time, highlighting those areas where you feel you need the most improvement. Mark up each chapter with plenty of notes, indicating possible strategies you feel you could best use to change your current routine or lifestyle. You may skim over topics that you feel you are already strong in or that don't really apply to you. Then, after reading this book the first time, go through it once again, focusing on the highlighted areas and notes you have marked or jotted down.

Create Lifestyle Changes for the Better

Changing up the way you go about your day can be quite challenging, no doubt. It may also seem to you that the older you are, the more set in your ways you've become. You may feel that making drastic changes in your diet, exercise regimen, and other realms of your life is more difficult with age. After all, you are facing a change in the way you live your life. Whether it is for the better or not, it's still quite a task to make any major lifestyle alterations.

So often you may see others who have tried to make simple alterations in their daily regimens but failed. You may wonder if making a change for the long term is really practical. Most people have no idea what they are getting into when they make such commitments to themselves.

What you must realize before jumping into a resolution is that you are going up against a lifetime of habits. You must recognize the need for a change and what's in it for you both in the short term and in the long term, and ultimately, accept that you have some work to do in accomplishing such changes for a better you.

Once you make a decision to change a certain aspect of your lifestyle, attaining your goal is that much easier. Just bear in mind that you must keep your goal at a high priority, with solid commitment and awareness for the long term. Devise a strategy and stick to it. If you do these things, making a healthy lifestyle change will become much easier.

Contents

CHAPTER 1

YOU ARE WHAT YOU EAT

YOU'VE HEARD THIS saying before. Supporting your body's billions of cells begins with the nutrition you're feeding those cells. Great nutrition leads to healthy, robust cells and better overall bodily functions. Your body is in many ways a product of what foods you feed it. There are many nutrients in the foods we eat—some of which are antioxidants, which aid the body in fighting off free radicals (including cancerous cells) and thus improve one's immune system and help prevent wrinkles, gray hair, and other aging traits. Foods also contain protein, carbohydrates, and fats; these are referred to as macronutrients. These macronutrients house the energy (measured in kilocalories) that is needed to fuel your body for general function. Certain foods are more nutrient-dense than others. Your goal is to include more foods with a high density of antioxidant nutrients. Most of these power-packed, antioxidant-rich foods can be found in the produce section of your local grocery store.

When you shop at the grocery store, remember this little tip: most of your shopping should be done around the perimeter of the supermarket. Only occasionally should you be picking up items from the aisles in the grocery store. Think about it: where is the produce section in most stores? Where are the fresh meat and seafood located? And please stay away from the candy, snack, and bread aisles. Avoid the bakery section altogether.

When you go grocery shopping, go on a full stomach. Never shop for groceries when you're hungry. It's funny how you might not even like blueberry pie all that much, but if you see one while passing by the bakery section, and you haven't eaten anything all day, you suddenly think it's a good idea to place the pie in your shopping cart. We've all been there; you know exactly what I'm talking about. So my advice to you is, if you're ever going to indulge and overeat, doing it just before grocery shopping would be the ideal time.

The Cornerstones of a Healthy Diet

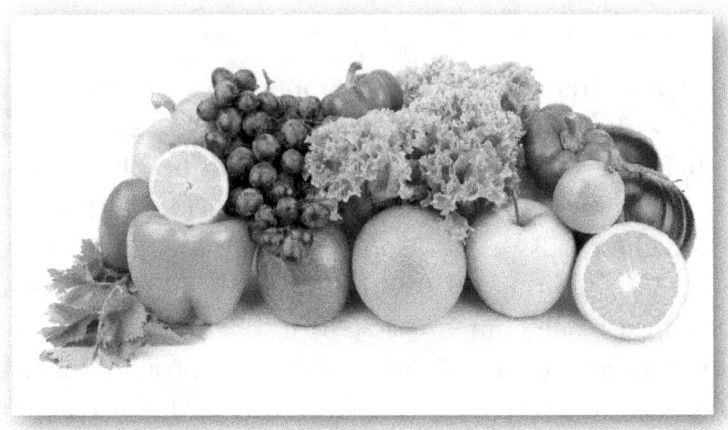

Dark Green Leaves

Dark green leafy vegetables are widely known for their high antioxidant density, so the addition of this class of vegetable is paramount in the antiaging diet. High intake of such nutrient-rich green vegetables has been associated with lower risks of cancer—especially lung, colon, prostate, and breast cancers.

Kale

When you look for power-packed foods with the greatest bang for the bite, there may be no greater food on the planet than kale. Rightfully referred to by many as the "queen of greens," this leaf is ultra-low in calories, high in fiber, and has zero grams of fat. But that's hardly scratching the surface as to why this is such an excellent staple food for your anti-aging diet. Beyond aiding in digesting and eliminating food due to its high fiber content, kale is loaded with nutrients such as magnesium, folate, sulfur, calcium, iron, vitamin A, vitamin C, vitamin K, lutein, and other antioxidants such as carotenoids and flavonoids that help fight cancer cells.

The addition of kale in the diet may help improve your cardiovascular function due to the lowering of cholesterol levels. The power leaf is also a great anti-inflammatory food. Just one cup of kale contains 10 percent of the recommended daily allowance of omega-3 fatty acids, which may help with arthritis, asthma, various autoimmune conditions, and other inflammatory conditions.

Spinach

Another power food in the dark-green leafy veggie category is spinach. Popeye's favorite food is certainly power-packed, containing antioxidants such as vitamin A, vitamin C, folic acid, lutein, and carotenoids. Even though virtually all vegetables contain a wide variety of phytonutrients such as flavonoids and carotenoids, spinach ranks among the highest in phytonutrient content. Studies have shown that spinach contains more than a dozen variations of flavonoid compounds, which are known to have anti-inflammatory and anticancer properties.

CRUCIFEROUS VEGETABLES

Another class of nutrient-dense vegetable is the cruciferous family. Cruciferous vegetables include broccoli, brussel sprouts, bok choy, cabbage, cauliflower, collard greens, horseradish, maca, mustard greens, radish, and turnips. They are rich in vitamins, minerals, phytochemicals, and fiber—much like the dark-green leafy veggies. They, too, are popular for their anti-cancer and anti-inflammatory properties, being nutrient-dense and full of antioxidants (like kale and spinach).

This family of vegetables is also low in calories, high in nutrients, high in fiber, and has practically zero fat. This group of veggies must also be a staple in one's anti-aging diet. The strong smell and bitter taste of cruciferous vegetables are due to a sulfur compound, known as phenylthiocarbamide. Depending on the genotype of the taster, most people will taste the bitterness of cruciferous veggies.

Dark green and cruciferous vegetables are in a league of their own when it comes to nutrient-density and age-defying properties. These foods should be your main source of fuel if you are looking to stay healthy and lean and maintain youthful-looking skin. If you want to be youthful now and for years to come, don't go a day without at least two servings of these superfoods.

BERRIES
Berries—such as blueberries, blackberries, cranberries, strawberries, and raspberries—are very high in antioxidants such as anthocyanins and flavonols. These substances protect against cellular damage and therefore aid in fighting off free radicals that could bring on diabetes and cancer. Berries are also full of vitamin C, which helps to repair damaged skin and other tissues and helps to prevent skin cancer.

Darker berries, such and blackberries and blueberries, contain the most antioxidants of any berries. Simply adding one serving of these berries per day will greatly benefit your goal of slowing down the aging process.

Acai Berries
The acai berry has been touted as a superfood, as it is known for aiding digestion, improving energy, strengthening the immune system, and helping the heart, not to mention assisting with anti-aging and weight loss. Indeed, the acai berry has high-antioxidant content—which may help with immune system function, energy improvement, and anti-aging factors—and high fiber—which helps in digestion. However, there is very little research to back up claims that the berry produces any true weight loss benefits. Nevertheless, this is indeed a fruit to add to your diet, with all of its oxidation-fighting goodness.

Pomegranate
In ancient times, pomegranate was actually used for medicinal purposes. Our ancestors were on to something, no doubt. This superfood is

loaded with antioxidants, including such phytochemicals as tannins and anthocyanins. These phytochemicals guard against cancer cell replication, help prevent the development of arteriosclerosis, and improve the look and feel of your skin.

Due to its high vitamin C content, pomegranate improves skin suppleness by hydrating the skin. It helps replenish dry skin cells and softens the skin via an internal mechanism when taken orally, or externally when applied as a cream or gel containing pomegranate.

FRUITS

There has been a lot of confusion as to which fruits are good for you and which are less-than-stellar food choices. Fruits are all nutritious in their own respective qualities. However, some are very high on the glycemic scale (i.e., they raise your blood sugar). Fruits such as berries, apples, pomegranates, and plums are great choices because of their high fiber content. It is the fiber that lowers the glycemic-index rating, as fiber essentially negates the impact of sugar intake when it comes to spiking your blood sugar and insulin release.

Fruits that score somewhere in the middle on the glycemic index are OK to be taken in moderation (one serving a day). One note to remember is that it's better to consume foods that will significantly raise your blood sugar level in the early part of the day so you'll have time during your active day to burn off the circulating glucose in the blood. For this reason, you may want to include these in your breakfast or mid-day meal. Examples of these fruits are bananas, oranges, pears, and kiwifruit.

Now for the fruits that should be limited in your anti-aging diet. These fruits significantly raise blood sugar levels, as they are at the top of the glycemic index. Examples are melons, pineapple, grapes, dates, and apricots. These have relatively little fiber and very high sugar content. That's not a good combination when your goal is to keep your blood sugar levels, and your insulin levels, at a steady state throughout the day.

Insulin Spikes and Aging

Why do we need to worry about what spikes our insulin levels? A spike in blood sugar and an increase in the secretion of insulin from the pancreas create a cascade of events in the body. This cascade includes the release of certain hormones into the bloodstream, resulting in the tearing down of various body tissues such as muscle fibers, collagen in the skin, and so forth, and the shuttling of energy molecules from food (glucose that is converted to fat) into the body's fat stores. We will explain this reaction to increased blood sugar further when we go over the reasons for practicing proper meal-portion control, with the aim of slowing your body's aging processes.

Eat More Fish

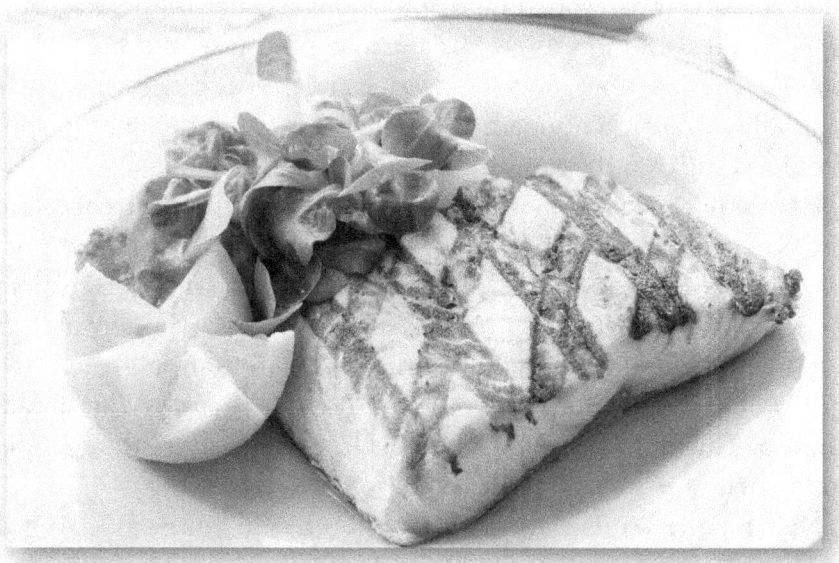

You have probably been told that fish is good for you so many times that you considered bypassing this discussion. The reason for its fame is that it contains essential fatty acids (not all fish). The omega-3 fatty acids in certain types of fish have tremendous benefits to your health and are key components in a diet geared toward anti-aging.

There is ample evidence to support that the oils in darker-colored fish—such as salmon, tuna, herring, and mackerel—are beneficial for the heart and brain and may even lower the risk of cancer. Fish oils are also positively linked to improved skin health, weight loss and weight management, cholesterol levels, triglyceride levels, and to some extent, blood sugar levels. Omega-3s found in fish may also be of some benefit in protecting against memory loss.

Eating salmon is one of the best ways to get healthy omega-3 fatty acids in your diet because of its high fat content. According to acclaimed dermatologist Nicholas Perricone (author of *The Wrinkle Cure),* the regular consumption of foods high in omega-3 fatty acids positively correlates with a reduction in the body's production of inflammatory compounds.[i] Such inflammatory compounds hasten the aging of the body's tissues, and therefore have a negative impact on the integrity, suppleness, and overall health of the skin.

You should have at least two 3-ounce servings of fish each week. Remember this, though: don't just eat any type of fish. The fish should be wild-caught, as most farm-raised fish are lacking in omega-3 content in comparison to any wild-caught fish. Also, try sticking to the darker types of fish, as I mentioned earlier.

Nuts and Seeds

Don't be fooled by the fact that nuts and seeds are calorie-dense and contain high amounts of fat. The fat in them are just the kind you want—healthy unsaturated fats, mostly monounsaturated, which are great for your heart and blood vessels. They are good sources of protein and fiber, and contain plant sterols and stanols, which have powerful cholesterol-lowering properties. Most nuts and seeds contain antioxidants such as vitamin E, all of the B vitamins, and several essential minerals.

The healthiest of the bunch in this food group is the walnut. Walnuts are high in omega-3 fatty acids as well as the minerals manganese and copper. They also contain essential amino acids, which the body needs in order to produce nitric oxide, a chemical responsible for the elasticity and pliability of blood vessels.

Other great choices for nuts and seeds include almonds, Brazil nuts, flaxseeds, pumpkin seeds, sunflower seeds, and sesame seeds. It would be ideal to include a variety of these nuts and seeds in a snack or small meal, as each of these has its own unique blend of vitamins, minerals, essential amino acids, and essential fatty acids.

GREEK YOGURT

Greek yogurt has several unique benefits for the body. One cup of low-fat Greek yogurt has more calcium than one cup of low-fat milk, with nearly three times the amount of protein compared to low-fat milk. This makes Greek yogurt a very important contributor to the health of your bones, muscles, tendons, and ligaments, and quite helpful in healing tissues throughout the body.

The difference between traditional yogurt and Greek yogurt is that Greek yogurt has been strained to remove the whey. As a result, Greek yogurt is creamier, thicker, and richer in flavor than traditional yogurt. The removal of whey results in a healthier yogurt with 40 percent less sugar, 35 percent less sodium, and more than twice the amount of protein in comparison to traditional yogurt.[ii]

Greek yogurt is also helpful for digestive health. It has a high content of probiotics, which are healthy bacteria that promote a healthy environment in the small intestine. It is the small intestine that is responsible for the majority of food digestion and nutrient absorption into the bloodstream, for delivery of nutrients to all tissues of the body.

The small intestine contains many types of bacteria; some are good, helping you digest food, and some are potentially harmful. Consuming probiotics such as those found in Greek yogurt helps increase the percentage and number of healthy bacteria in your digestive tract. As a result, this leaves less room for the unhealthy bacteria of the small intestine to thrive and grow. Maintaining such a healthy balance of healthy bacteria to unhealthy bacteria may help keep you regular, as the good bacteria will fight off the bad bacteria that commonly cause diarrhea. Probiotics may also be helpful for people suffering from irritable bowel syndrome or from intestinal diseases such as Crohn's disease and ulcerative colitis. For ideas on how to include Greek yogurt into your diet, I recommend you read *The Greek Yogurt Kitchen: More Than 130 Delicious, Healthy Recipes for Every Meal of the Day.*[iii] In this book, renowned dietitian Toby Amidor explains the value of adding this healthful food item to your diet, while laying out many tasty ideas for its inclusion.

It is also important to note that Greek yogurt does not need to be omitted from your diet if you are lactose intolerant. If you are lactose intolerant, you should still keep some amounts of dairy products in your diet, according to recommendations by the National Institutes of Health and the National Medical Association.

Studies have found that people with lactose intolerance can tolerate up to one cup of milk per meal, which contains twelve grams of lactose. For those who are lactose intolerant, it is recommended that you start introducing lactose slowly into your diet and begin with lower lactose-containing foods such as Greek yogurt. A six-ounce container of nonfat plain Greek yogurt contains only four grams of lactose, making this a safe product for you even if you are lactose intolerant.

Portion Control

It is important that you learn to properly control the portions of your meals. Smaller-sized meals scattered throughout the day are far more beneficial to your health that one, two, or even three larger meals. For one, regular snacks keep the body fed on a consistent basis, rather than going through a cycle of hunger and gorging. Your metabolism will increase if your body is fed calories via small amounts of food at times that are spread evenly throughout the day, rather than from just a couple large meals in the day. After all, as mammals we are designed to be grazers.

A review published in a 2003 edition of the *American Journal of Clinical Nutrition* concludes that restriction in caloric intake results in lower metabolic rate and oxidative stress in animals.[iv] This reduction in oxidative stress lowers the body's secretion of stress hormones such as cortisol, which contributes to the breakdown (and aging) of various tissues in the body.

Therefore, the takeaway from the linkage between caloric intake and aging is that eating less food at a given sitting may result in less stress hormone in the body. In contrast, the consumption of high-calorie meals will encourage the body to release higher amounts of stress hormones, which may accelerate the aging of tissues.

As far as the correct size of the portion for a given food or meal, there is a simple estimation method to use as a guide. You can associate food items with other objects. For example, a single cup of pasta or rice is about the size of a tennis ball. A healthy-sized portion of fish or chicken should be three to four ounces, which is the size of a deck of cards.

The amount of food you consume has an effect on blood sugar, particularly if you are diabetic. Eating larger portions than your body requires is sure to raise your blood sugar levels. Although foods with carbohydrates have the largest impact on blood sugars, eating too much of any type of food will cause blood sugar spikes, and in effect, weight gain.

Eating smaller portions four or five times a day is important for more reasons than reducing your waistline. Overeating has been linked to nerve cell death in the brain, according to a research study by endocrinologist Zane Andrews.[v] His study concluded that free radicals attacked neurons in the brain after subjects had eaten a meal. This destruction of brain cells was further increased when the subjects consumed carbohydrates and sugars.

What is worse for jolting your blood sugar level than eating a large meal? Eating foods that have a high glycemic-index rating. Some of these foods may surprise you. For instance, a potato sounds like a healthy food to many. It is a great source of vitamin C, and has plenty of potassium as well as several B vitamins. It's considered a vegetable. It doesn't taste sweet at all, really. However, a potato has the same glycemic index rating as table sugar! Then you have pastas, breads (wheat bread included), and many other foods that many of us would not consider to taste sweet, yet are scoring eighty or higher on the glycemic-index chart.

LIVING HEALTHY WITH DIABETES

If you're a diabetic, there are a few more hurdles you will have to jump over when it comes to living a healthy life and slowing the aging process. Diabetes can lead to degeneration of nervous tissue if your blood sugar is not well maintained. Diabetics who do not properly maintain their blood sugar levels may end up suffering from nerve-degenerating disorders such as macular degeneration in the eyes and diabetic peripheral neuropathy in the feet and legs. Due to this nerve degeneration, diabetics are at risk for major complications from slow wound healing, which could conceivably result in the amputation of a limb.

While it is true we cannot control our genetic makeup, age, or family history of diabetes, there is much we can control that affects whether we develop type 2 diabetes on the one hand, or whether the disease gets worse on the other hand. If you are a diabetic or have a genetic predisposition for diabetes, you can take steps to maximize your health potential, add years to your life, and improve your quality of life during those added years. Steps to take to stay at your healthiest as a diabetic include the following:

- Live a healthier lifestyle through a low-glycemic and well-balanced diet, exercising properly, and quitting smoking if you currently smoke.
- Keep track of your blood sugar, blood pressure, cholesterol, and weight. These numbers tell you how well your diabetes is being managed.
- Don't miss your doctor's appointments. Also be sure to follow your doctor's orders. With diabetes, several aspects of health may be affected, such as your vision, your feet and legs, and your heart. For this reason, you may have several healthcare professionals observing and treating you for your condition.

If you're like most diabetics, you may be constantly asking yourself, "What can I eat?" or "What must I cut out of my diet?" Fortunately, living with diabetes doesn't mean you have to feel deprived. While you should avoid sugars and starchy carbohydrates as much as you can, there are many food choices that may satisfy your sweet tooth without significantly affecting your blood sugar.

- Berries are loaded in fiber, have a low glycemic-index (GI) rating, and have a lot of antioxidants.
- Apples and oranges are low-GI fruits as well.
  - Avoid high-sugar fruits such as melons, pineapple, and grapes. The glycemic indices of these fruits are so high that they will affect your blood sugar levels as much as eating pure table sugar.
- Sweet potatoes are considered low on the glycemic index and are a good choice as low-impact carbohydrate food. Have this in place of regular potatoes as a lower- GI alternative.
- Whole grains are a great low-GI food. This is because of the germ and the bran in the grains. Germ and bran contain all the nutrients a grain product has to offer. When you eat processed grains like bread made from enriched wheat flour, you don't get the germ and bran. In the absence of these important ingredients, you lose the fiber; therefore, your blood sugar levels will go up with the consumption of processed grains.

There are many foods that are satisfying and can help you avoid overeating. Low-calorie and high-fiber veggies, nuts, and omega-3–rich fish are all great choices for this.

- Nuts are good for diabetics because there is very little sugar in them, plus they have protein, healthy fats, vitamins, and minerals that are important for your body. The healthy fats in them also help with satiety.
- Dark-green, leafy vegetables, such as kale, spinach, and collard, are the most antioxidant-rich foods on the planet. They also have practically no effect on your blood sugar when you eat them. Eat all you want of these—the more the better.

- Salmon is the most popular of the fish that are high in omega-3 fatty acids. The health benefits from this essential fatty acid, along with the high fat content (healthy fat) that is in salmon, make this fish a great food choice for diabetics, as well as anybody else, for both nutrition and satiety purposes.

As you can see from the foods to include and foods to avoid, as well as the lifestyle alterations that diabetics should work on, the changes a diabetic must make are not all that different from the changes that a nondiabetic must make to be healthy and feel young. This is the silver lining to living with diabetes—the recommended diet for you if you're a diabetic or at risk of developing diabetes is basically the same as it should be even if you do not have diabetes. If you just wanted to eat healthier, be more active, avoid many of the pitfalls of aging, and live better, the lifestyle of being a diabetic just might help and is really no different from a lifestyle focused on living healthy.

DRINK MORE WATER

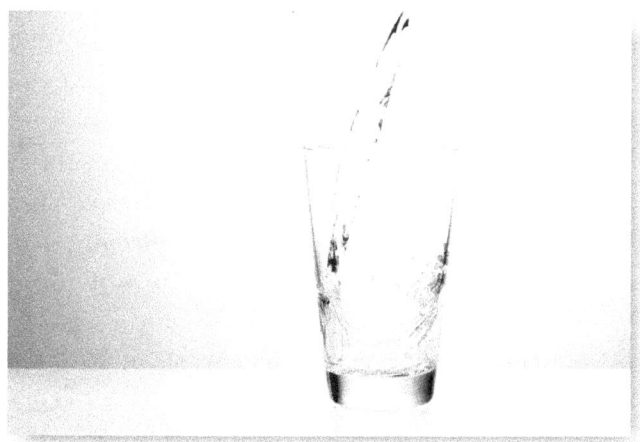

With approximately 60 percent of our bodies consisting of water, it is not difficult to understand why water is the single most important nutrient of all. Water is essential for your body's functions in a multitude of ways.

More water will not only flush out toxins and keep you hydrated for better organ function, but it is also a natural appetite suppressor and helps the body metabolize fat. To understand water's role in metabolizing fat, you will need to understand the basics of how the kidneys and the liver function.

When the kidneys don't get enough water, they are not able to function properly, so the liver is then required to take on the role of eliminating toxins from our bodies. Normally, one of the liver's major functions is to metabolize stored body fat into a usable form of energy. However, when the liver is occupied in taking over the kidneys' role in clearing out toxins from the body, it is less apt to metabolize the stored body fat. Then, as increasing fat is stored in the body, the ability for weight loss comes to a halt.

We need to keep ourselves properly hydrated for many other equally important reasons as well, as proper hydration is critical for preventing joint pain and inflammation, sustaining optimal cardiovascular function, enabling satiety and thus weight loss, and improving skin suppleness and radiance. Let's look at other ways in which increased water consumption helps with our overall health, vitality, and anti-aging.

JOINT HEALTH
If you have joint pain that is not due to gout, arthritis, or the flu, there is a good chance it could be the result of dehydration. While increasing your water consumption may not cure your joint pain, it may certainly help with hydration of the joints, which will help with joint lubrication, and therefore, may decrease pain associated with osteoarthritis. A viscous liquid substance that is secreted within all movable joints of your body, known as synovial fluid, is primarily made up of water, along with hyaluronic acid (which makes up the viscous aspect of this fluid) and other nutrients. Without the adequate secretion of this fluid within the inner membranes of your joints, there is increased friction within the

joint articulation, between the coating of cartilage that exists between the bones. This friction is basically the direct rubbing together of the cartilage coatings over the bones within the joints (or in severe cases, with cartilage withered away due to chronic degenerative changes, the direct rubbing of the bones together). Such friction will cause discomfort with movement.

If a joint is healthy and well-nourished via proper secretion of synovial fluid, it will be able to move without pain, given there are no other underlying conditions. Such conditions may include buildup of acidic crystals, an injury to the tissues within the joint, or chronic degenerative changes within the joint articulation.

CARDIOVASCULAR HEALTH

There is ample evidence suggesting that properly hydrating your body is an effective action against the development or progression of heart disease. A research study published in a 2002 edition of the *American Journal of Epidemiology* demonstrated a high correlation between improved daily intake of water and a decreased risk of coronary artery disease in both men and women. The researchers in this study noted more viscosity of the blood, more volume of red blood cells, and more clotting proteins among subjects who consumed less than two glasses of water a day, relative to the individuals in the study who drank five or more.[vi]

An elevation in blood viscosity, or blood thickness, is associated with coronary artery disease. Elevated hematocrit, fibrinogen, and blood viscosity are indicators that are actually found years prior to the symptoms of cardiovascular conditions coming to the surface, and as such, are used as markers for a patient who is at risk for future coronary artery disease. With thicker blood comes decreased speed of blood flow in the arteries. This then leads to clots, arteriosclerosis (hardening of the walls of the arteries), and high blood pressure. The simplest lifestyle change in fighting against this elevated blood thickness and destruction of the endothelial walls within your arteries is drinking plenty of water to keep yourself well-hydrated.

WEIGHT LOSS

Weight loss plans should really be focusing more heavily on the consumption of water throughout the day. A study presented by Dr. Brenda Davy at the 2010 National Meeting of the American Chemical Society in Boston held that people who consumed two cups of water before a meal were shaving 75 to 95 percent off the calories that the meal would have represented had they not drunk the two cups of water.[vii]

The science behind this decrease in appetite while drinking plenty of water is quite simple. The fact that good old water is calorie-free is one reason. Another obvious reason is that drinking a sufficient amount of water will fill the stomach up. Satiety will be achieved more easily when you include a couple eight-ounce glasses of water with your meal. This is particularly true if you drink sixteen ounces of water just prior to eating your meal, as opposed to sipping your water throughout the meal.

The bottom line: if your drink more water before beginning your meal, your desire for eating will be lessened. The result will be more calorie-free, detoxifying water drunk and less food consumed.

SKIN HEALTH

Adequate water consumption for the body is essential in maintaining skin moisture, as it is needed for the delivery of essential nutrients to the skin cells. No one wants dry, dehydrated skin. Dehydrated skin gives the obvious and unsightly attributes we all want to avoid: flakiness, tightness, and roughness of skin.

Dry skin is more prone to wrinkling, as it has less elasticity. In order to have soft, moist skin, the importance of drinking an adequate amount of water daily far outweighs the need to apply lotion to the skin every day. The intake of water takes care of the hydration of the skin cells from within. Not that you shouldn't work on your skin from the outside as well—that also has its place. We will discuss the necessity for skin creams and lotions in more detail in a later chapter.

How Much Water Should You Drink Each Day?

The National Academy of Sports Medicine recommends ninety-six ounces of water per day. This is twelve eight-ounce glasses of water. To many, this sounds like an incredible, or even unattainable, amount of water to take in within a twenty-four-hour period, but it really isn't.

If you absolutely cannot stand to drink water, there are ways to make this task of increasing your water intake more enjoyable. Simply adding a lemon or lime in with your glass of water may make it easier to down the water. There are several powdered beverage mixes on the market that will also make drinking water more palatable. Just remember to watch the calories you are adding to the water, so you don't negate the benefits of drinking more water in the first place.

Detoxifying Cleanses

Detoxifying cleanses have been around for centuries, used then for the same reasons that they are used today. To detoxify your body, you must focus on resting, cleansing, and nourishing your body from within. Such cleanses for removing toxins can help you to have more energy, boost your immune system, lose weight, clear up certain digestive problems, decrease muscle and joint aches, and allow for healthier-looking skin and hair, among other benefits. If you have any of the following, you should strongly consider a detox cleanse:

- bloating
- sluggishness or unexplained fatigue
- unexplained muscle and joint aches
- irritated skin
- mental confusion
- menstrual problems
- often having low-grade infections
- puffiness or dark shadiness under the eyes

When detoxing, you are essentially cleaning the blood by removing impurities from the blood in the liver, which is where toxins are processed for elimination. Other organs involved in toxin elimination are the kidneys, intestines, lungs, lymph, and skin. When your system for eliminating toxins is compromised, impurities are no longer filtered properly, causing your body's organs and tissues to be negatively affected.

Detox programs target the body's toxins at the cellular level. As naturopathic physician Peter Bennett, coauthor of *7-Day Detox Miracle*, explains, "Detoxification works because it addresses the needs of individual cells, the smallest units of human life."[viii] Purifying the body at this level will set your body's organs up for much better function.

A detox program will naturally help cleanse the body in a few ways. First, the detox allows organs to have a "break," so they are not working extra-hard due to the toxin buildup in the cells. Also, the detox stimulates the liver to pull more toxins from the body, while also promoting toxin elimination through the intestines, kidneys, and skin. Finally, the detox program will allow for the refueling of healthy nutrients for the cells of the body after the "dumping" of so much of your cells' toxins.

There are many detox cleanses out there, but some of the most widely known categories are juice or smoothie cleanses, sugar detox, colon cleanses, and hypoallergenic detox. They all have different benefits and fit the needs of each person differently. Many cleanse programs span about seven to ten days, giving the time necessary for cleaning the blood. I personally recommend a seven-day juice fast—where you are to only drink water and fresh fruit and vegetable juices, along with some walnuts or almonds for healthy fats and protein—for an entire week. I have tried this before by taking in only purified water, organic kale, blueberries, blackberries, and raspberries for seven days. I can say that my energy levels soared after the cleanse, as did my clarity of thinking.

Dr. Mote's Seven-Day Detox Diet:

Using a Vitamix blender, I fill the blender from one-half to three-quarters full of organic kale, then adding one and a half to two cups of frozen berries (organic blueberries, raspberries, and blackberries), and two cups of water. This is for breakfast, lunch, and dinner for the next seven days. I also have a handful of organic walnuts or almonds two to three times a day, spread out in between the smoothies. I sometimes also add a handful of these nuts in with the smoothies, for added protein and healthy fats.

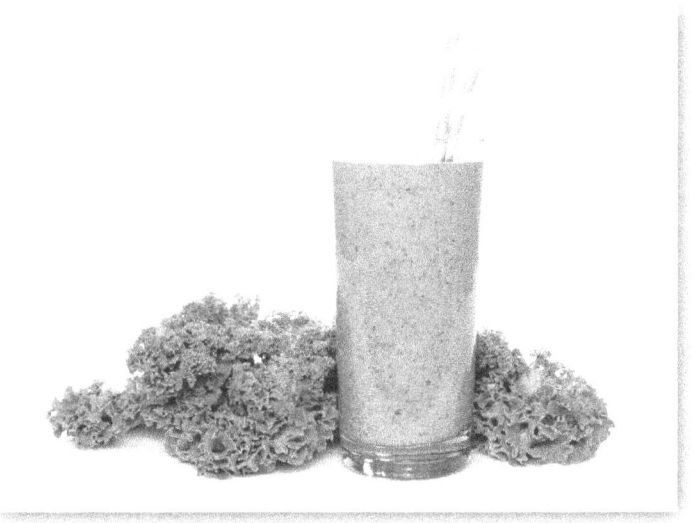

So a detoxification program is important and should be considered by anybody, as we all have toxins floating around in our bodies and stuck inside our tissues' cells. The following are practices you should take to cleanse your body:

- Drink at least one gallon of water a day.
- Take in lots of vitamin C—up to two thousand mg, preferably spread out throughout the day. This helps the body produce

glutathione, which is a liver compound that helps rid the body of toxins.

- Reduce negative stresses in your life as much as you can. For instance, worrying about things that are out of your control accomplishes nothing, other than diminishing your health.
- Go to the sauna regularly, as you can eliminate toxins through your sweat.
- Exercise in some way every day. One hour of some exhilarating activity—such as walking, jogging, swimming, weight training, yoga, Pilates, and so forth—has a positive effect on the body.

CHAPTER 2

EXERCISE-YOUR PRESCRIPTION FOR ANTI-AGING

IT IS NO secret that exercise is good for your health. For helping you to lose or manage your weight, to strengthen your muscles and bones, and to raise your endorphins and make you feel better, it's tough to beat exercise for engendering a healthy, active, and longer life. Several studies have found that exercise can be at least as effective as prescription drugs in preventing common health conditions such as heart disease, stroke, and diabetes.

It seems there is an endless list of reasons to exercise. It's really like a wonder drug, aiming at the prevention of several conditions and diseases, without any side effects. Let's explore some benefits of exercise.

BENEFITS OF EXERCISE

A GREAT WAY TO DE-STRESS

Stress is one of the worst enemies to your health, and consequently, it promotes aging. Cortisol is released (which wreaks havoc on the body in so many ways, as discussed earlier), you will have less sleep, and your cognition is no longer functioning at 100 percent. Regular exercise fights against stress by releasing endorphins, which give you that "runner's high" feeling. With sufficient exercise or invigorating activity, endorphins are secreted, and one's mood is elevated. Working out will also help you get your mind off the things that are stressing you out so much.

There's no better de-stressor than redirecting your focus on to exhilarating physical activity—perhaps jogging, lifting weights, or running sprints. My personal favorite is sprint interval training, a form of high-intensity interval training. We'll say more about this type of training later on in this chapter. With intense exercise activity, such as sprints, you will find you have a hard time focusing on anything other than getting through the workout. This is perfect if you want to get your mind off stressors that bring you down mentally or emotionally.

LIFTING YOUR MOOD

Working out vigorously for thirty to forty-five minutes at least three times a week can reduce symptoms of depression about as effectively as antidepressants, according to studies.[ix-x] Most likely, exercise stimulates the growth of neurons in certain brain regions that are damaged by depression. Also, studies of animals have found that vigorous physical activity increases the production and secretion of molecules that improve the connectivity between neurons in the brain, thus emulating the effects of antidepressants. Gamma-aminobutyric acid, commonly known as GABA, a brain chemical that is known for improving mood and decreasing anxiety, has also been shown in studies to increase with regular exercise.

Interval training is the best way to get the euphoric "runner's high" feeling. This may be performed with sprint bursts in running, biking, or swimming, where you perform the activity as fast as you can for thirty to forty-five seconds, followed by rest or reduced speed for two to three minutes, and repeating this for five to ten times. GABA production is just one of the many great benefits of interval training.

BUILDING YOUR CONFIDENCE

Noticing even small improvements in your fitness, such as your ability to run an extra mile or adding more weight to the bar in the gym, gives you a self-esteem surge. When you begin to see actual changes in your physical appearance as a result of working out, your confidence level gets an even greater boost. If you are far from your goal aesthetically, take before-and-after photos to reveal your progress. Start by taking pictures of yourself now, without clothes on, and again one week later. It is not so easy for you to see changes by looking into the mirror every day, as the changes are so subtle. But one week of changes can be significant. When you see these results for yourself, giving you visual proof of the effectiveness of all the effort you are putting into your diet and exercise, you will feel motivated to carry on and work to improve even further.

IMPROVE YOUR SLEEP

According to the National Sleep Foundation, there is ample evidence to support the idea that regular exercise has a positive effect on our sleep. [xi] When you work out, you burn calories and expend energy. This transfers to an increased need for your body to sleep, which reenergizes you for the next day. You will, however, need to avoid working out within two to three hours of bedtime, or the exercise will actually have a negative effect on sleeping by keeping you awake due to the elevated levels of endorphins, heart rate, and blood circulation.

When it comes to receiving the benefits of improved sleep, the best time to exercise would be in the morning. This is because you expend a great amount of energy with your morning blast, energizing you for hours thereafter and kick-starting your day; as the day goes on, your energy steadily decreases, priming you for better rest by nighttime. Another good time to work out (for improved sleep) would be around noon or early afternoon—perhaps during your lunch break on a workday. Just remember, whatever time you work out, make sure it's not within two hours of bedtime.

MORE ENERGY THROUGHOUT THE DAY

Working out is a great way to energize yourself for the rest of the day, while helping you rest much better at the end of the day. Ideally, working out around lunchtime is a great way to boost your energy levels that naturally start to taper off around early afternoon. Working out in the morning is also great, but many morning exercisers notice too much of a decline in energy by two or three o'clock in the afternoon.

Boost Your Immune System
Exercise boosts your body's immune function, decreasing your chances of getting sick. Some studies suggest that people with a regular exercise regimen are about half as likely to contract a common cold as those who do not work out regularly.

Improve Your Life Expectancy
Exercise can significantly improve your life expectancy. Some researchers have found that regular exercise can increase your life-span as much as stopping smoking—by about seven years. If you currently live a sedentary lifestyle, sitting at a desk all day, or lying on the couch for six or more hours a day, you have a 64 percent increased risk of dying from heart disease, as well as a higher risk for certain types of cancer. So get moving—your life depends on it.

Improve Your Mind
With regular exercise, you will think more clearly, retain information better, and have better mental focus. Exercise is perhaps the best medicine of all in terms of improving memory, mood, and cognition.

A thirty-minute stint of vigorous exercise will increase levels of serotonin, dopamine, and norepinephrine—chemicals in the brain involved in positive mood and better cognitive function. Exercise may actually work on a cellular level to reverse the impact stress has had on your aging process, according to a 2010 study from the University of California at San Francisco. The study discovered that highly stressed women who engaged in vigorous exercise for approximately forty-five minutes over a three-day period had fewer signs of aging in their cells compared to women who were living with comparably high levels of stress without exercising.[xii]

When you exercise, you are also improving your ability to learn by increasing the production and secretion of growth factors. These are chemicals that stimulate neuron growth and also improve connections between neurons in the brain, improving your learning and other cognitive skills. You improve these connections even more when you engage in an exercise that combines vigorous activity with coordination, such as tennis. With such an activity, you are essentially stressing your brain cells in order to stimulate them to grow, develop, and improve connectivity and information transmission. The same principle applies to muscle tissue—without added stress to the muscles, there will be no increase in growth. Conversely, just as not using a muscle leads to muscular atrophy, a lack of stimulation can lead to the degeneration and deterioration of nerve cells.

Just taking a leisurely walk for a mile or so a day can fight off memory loss and keep cognitive function strong in the elderly. In a 2011 study published in the *Archives of Internal Medicine,* elderly people who engaged in short walks, cooking, cleaning, and gardening were compared with other elders who were sedentary over the course of five years. The group that performed light activity retained more cognitive function than the sedentary group. In fact, 90 percent of the participants who performed light activity retained all of their cognitive capabilities at the end of the study period.[xiii]

There is also research showing that those who are genetically prone to Alzheimer's disease but nevertheless engage in some exercise are about four times less likely to suffer from the disease than those who are sedentary.

KEEP YOUR MUSCLES STRONG

Muscle strength is a prime component of healthy aging. As we age after our early forties, there is a slow, steady decline in muscle mass. It is no surprise that those who work out have more muscle mass than those in their age group who are sedentary. But even if you are not actually lifting weights, you are slowing the deterioration of your muscles by exercising. Any type of exercise that involves your body working against gravity will help build your muscles. Without regular exercise, however, your muscles will breakdown, resulting in muscle atrophy and decreased strength.

You should perform some type of weight-bearing exercise. If you are not all that excited about taking up weight lifting, using therapy bands, or doing resistance training to gain strength and muscle mass, you may alternatively engage in running, jumping rope, or dancing to keep your muscles strong.

Maintain Strong, Healthy Bones

We all lose bone density as we age. Just like with muscle mass, the deterioration of our bone density begins around our forties, and accelerates if we are sedentary. Exercise helps with this in the same way it helps with your muscles. If you are placing stress on the bones, your body reacts by stimulating osteoblasts, which are the cells in your bones that rebuild bone tissue. Exercise is not the only thing needed to maintain or improve bone density; calcium and vitamin D in the diet go hand in hand with exercise to complete the equation. You cannot have one or even two of the three and expect your bones to stay strong. All three have to be there: exercise, calcium, and vitamin D.

Lose Weight and Keep It Off

It comes as no surprise that most people work out to lose weight. Activity of any kind burns calories beyond what your body will burn at a resting state. The higher the intensity and duration of a round of exercise, the more calories you expend to fuel the efforts. The idea of working out seems to scare or confuse so many—those who struggle with weight wonder which mode of exercise is best for melting off the fat, how much or how little they should eat, how often they need to eat, and so on. Although there are subtle details as to which modes of exercise are best for shedding body fat and which are best for building muscle, the basis of weight loss and weight management remains unchanged—calories in versus calories out. If you are consuming fewer calories than your body is burning off, you are losing weight. If you eat more than you burn, you are going the opposite way. Too many people try to overcomplicate this.

The use of a device such as a Fitbit, Jawbone, Fuelband, or other gadgets that track activity performed throughout the day and measures your caloric expenditure is great for controlling your weight.

SAVE YOUR JOINTS WITH WEIGHT LOSS

Losing weight or maintaining a healthy body weight has the benefit of taking pressure off your joints, sparing them from early degeneration and breakdown. You may not realize it, but with every step you take throughout your life, the pressure on your joints will be made worse if you are carrying extra body weight. To carry even a single pound of extra body weight places added physical stress on the joints in your feet, ankles, knees, hips, and spine. The pressure is made worse if you are walking up or down steps, and much worse when running. The pressure on joints and on disc spaces in the spine is detrimental with a load heavier than the body is naturally designed to handle. The spine has to support much of the body's weight. Compression of intervertebral discs ensues, along with increased stress to the facet joints and to the supporting tissues of the spine. When seeing a patient dealing with back pain due to a compressed, bulging, or herniated disc, many medical doctors may tell the patient to lose weight, but at the same time he or she will write a prescription for an anti-inflammatory and send that patient out the door. Healthcare professionals realize that most people will struggle to shed their excess pounds. They also understand that most patients will not lose the excess weight for the long term. For this reason, it is much easier to medicate the condition rather than try to convince the patient that a lifestyle change is needed.

Joint arthrosis, known to most as arthritis, is stressful enough without adding the stress of losing weight to the equation. However, it is very important to find ways to shed the extra pounds, because with each minute you have that extra weight on you, increased joint compression is adding to your discomfort. Lose weight successfully and you will decrease much of the load on your joints. You will then be more open to dietary change and exercise, as the discomfort in exercise will be lessened with less body weight. By losing just a few pounds, your joints will have a greater chance of recovery. The joint arthrosis will progress considerably slower, your joints will receive a better nutrient supply through production of more synovial fluid, and the articular cartilage will last much longer.

Your joints have well-formed cartilage at youth, but through wear and tear, the articular cartilage is jeopardized. The result can be compared to metal rubbing against metal while the grease needed to lubricate the moving apparatus is worn away. Excess weight and reduced cartilage do a number on the knees—the articular cartilage diminishes, leading to increased inflammation and discomfort.

Unfortunately, arthritis will not resolve itself. As you age, you will only notice this worsen through increased wear and tear, if you neglect to take proper care of your joints. You can, indeed, slow its progression by taking certain actions. By losing weight, you can limit the forces exerted upon your joints as you go about your daily activities. Weight loss does involve making a few lifestyle changes, but drugs are not a requirement in your quest to lose the excess pounds. Losing weight and keeping it off is one aspect of control you can exert over the potentially incapacitating effects of joint arthrosis. Take control, get more active, lose weight, reduce your joint discomfort, and preserve the health of your joints.

Daily Activities of Today's World

Our bodies were genetically wired to be active. For so many of us who live sedentary lives, it should come as no surprise that we are seeing such a rise in obesity, diabetes, heart disease, and other concerning health complications. Such health conditions were much less prevalent in the days before desk jobs, desktops, mobile devices, and other modern bothers we have brought into our lives.

We have made our lives easy. We live in a time when our technology and ingenuity make it difficult for most of us to look back to the days before cars, television, and smartphones and understand how people could live without such conveniences. I find this reality to be rather dispiriting. We are a product of our environment. Our surroundings are filled with conveniences made to allow us to do less. Unfortunately, that means less physical activity. When you compound reduced physical activity with all of today's fast-food joints, processed foods, soda drinks, and so on, you can understand the rise in health insurance costs, the epidemic in obesity, and the trend of children developing adult-onset (type 2) diabetes.

Not all of today's conveniences doom us to inactivity, though. We are seeing a new age in gadgets, programs, and apps geared toward exercise and diet. We see fitness centers popping up more and more, in both urban and rural areas. The Internet can also be of great benefit in educating us on the countless methods of dieting, exercising, and living healthier.

Best Forms of Exercise

There are so many ways of exercising and engaging in activities that improve our health, there is little excuse for not participating in some type of moderate activity. By "moderate," I mean any activity you do that is the equivalent of a brisk walk. This could be doing yard work, cleaning your house, playing outside with your kids, and so on. There is no need to overcomplicate this matter—any activity is better than prolonged sitting or inactivity. If you currently live a sedentary lifestyle and the thought of exercising in any capacity scares you, start small by simply reducing your time sitting. Stand up and walk around at least once an hour for five minutes. Then soon begin going out for leisurely walks for fifteen to twenty minutes a day. After a week or two of light walking, move on to brisk walks. Don't go from zero to sixty by jumping right into high-intensity strength or cardio training if you're hardly used to leaving the sitting position every day.

Resistance Training

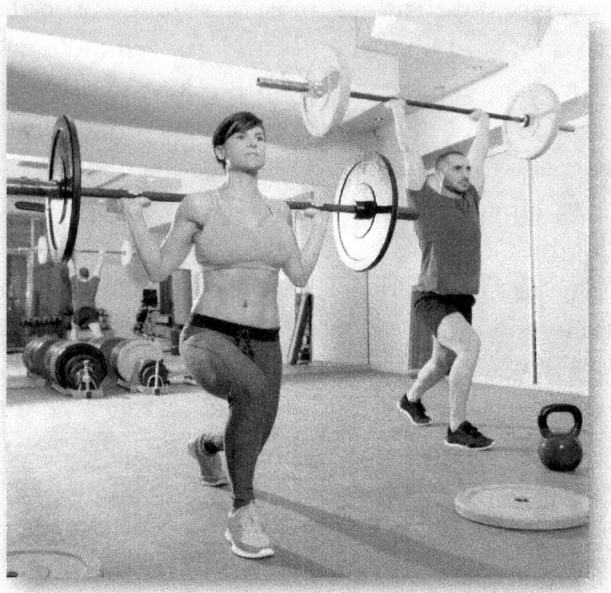

Resistance training is essential to a fitness routine; it helps build muscle mass while strengthening your bones as well. As we age after our thirties, strength training becomes more and more important, helping to offset the muscle and bone loss that occurs as a part of our natural aging process. Strength training can help increase muscle mass at any age.

Resistance training, also commonly referred to as strength training, helps in many ways:

- Lowering your blood sugar. As the muscle fibers work harder, more glycogen stores within the muscles are depleted, thus causing more absorption of glucose from the blood to replenish the glycogen stores, aiding the muscle tissue in recovery from exercise.
- Increasing your metabolism. Increased muscle mass causes the body to have a higher metabolic rate, as more calories are expended in a resting state with toned muscle.

- Strengthening your bones. Strength training increases bone density and reduces the risk of osteoporosis, as force on the bones causes more bone tissue to form in order to meet the higher demands.
- Improving your balance. Muscle strengthening contributes to improved balance, which is increasingly important as you age.

Resistance training does not have to be performed in the gym; you can engage in some form of resistance training in a swimming pool, at home in your living room, in a hotel room, in your bed, in a barn, or anywhere else for that matter. Here are some of the various modes of strength training:

- Free weights. Barbells and dumbbells are classic weight-training tools. Kettlebell weights are sometimes preferred over dumbbells, as kettlebell weights may allow for more versatility of movement.
- Weight machines. You will see resistance-training machines in most fitness centers, but there is also a large market for home weight machines. These machines are typically safe and convenient to use.
- Using your body weight. You can do many exercises with little or no equipment. Push-ups, pull-ups, abdominal crunches, walking lunges, and squats are all examples of strength-training exercises you can perform with much effectiveness with nothing more than your body weight.
- Resistance bands or tubing. Resistance bands and resistance tubing are inexpensive, lightweight tools that provide resistance when stretched. You can carry these bands or tubes anywhere. They are perfect for travelers who have little free time. There are countless exercises you can perform with these bands and tubes.

You will not need to spend hours a day lifting weights to reap the benefits of strength training. You need to spend only twenty to thirty minutes training, two to three times a week. Results are also noticed rather quickly from strength training. You will probably notice improvements in your strength and stamina in just two or three weeks, and will continue to see improvements as long as you are regularly exercising with resistance (regardless of your age).

CORE STRENGTHENING

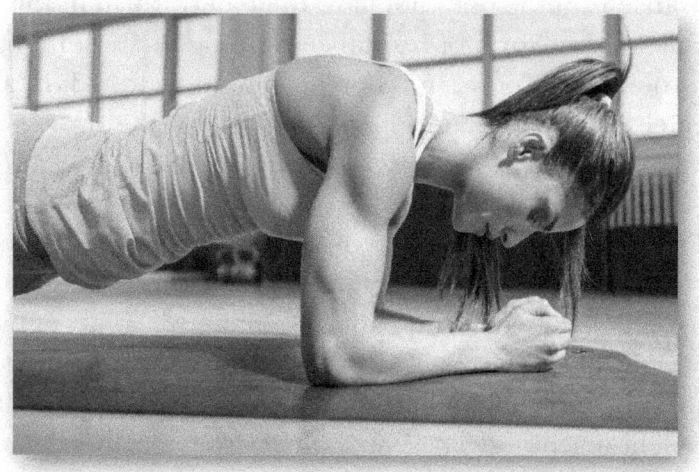

Another important aspect of strength training that needs to be mentioned is core strengthening. This is critical for preventing injuries, having better posture, improving in the performance of daily activities, not to mention advancing in one's athletic performance. Yet, as important as it may be, core strengthening and core stability training are so often neglected by even the most accomplished fitness buffs of the world. If you add this component into your regimen, whether you've worked out for years or are just thinking about starting, you will have an advantage that so few seem to grasp when it comes to improving overall physical function.

While everyone wants the supermodel body—chiseled abs and a statuesque rump—the benefits of a strong core reach far beyond aesthetics. And you don't have to purchase expensive equipment or join a gym to achieve core fitness.

Focused core strengthening that is aimed at training muscles in the hips, abdomen, lower back, and buttocks can boost your balance and stability, resulting in better physical performance on and off the field for athletes and better ergonomics for anybody.

If you are going for a firm, chiseled midsection, practicing targeted abdominal exercises, in combination with a regimen of aerobic training, is a good way to go. That is to say, aerobic activity burns abdominal fat while core exercises strengthen the underlying muscles.

Concentrated effort on strengthening one's core musculature can improve posture, balance, and flexibility, and even decrease or prevent back strains. Common core exercises include crunches, planks, and side bridges, but any exercise that uses the trunk of your body without the support of extremities qualifies as a core-strengthening exercise. Pilates is a form of training that I highly recommend for improving your core strength and stability. Even if you lift weights or work out regularly by other means, if you are new to Pilates, it is guaranteed to make you sore in the beginning. You will be working muscles you've never isolated before, in positions and ranges of motion that your muscles and joints are unaccustomed to. It will improve your overall fitness level by working on areas of your musculoskeletal system that you have unknowingly missed with other training.

FLEXIBILITY TRAINING

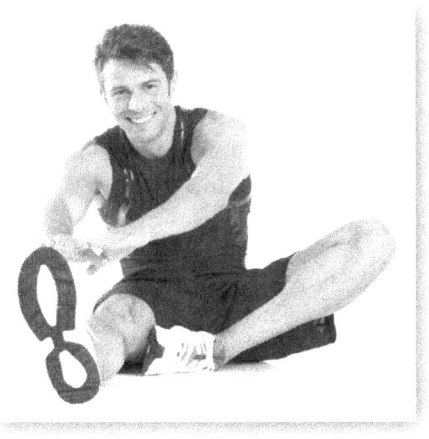

Flexibility training and strength training should go hand in hand, although this type of training is so often overlooked by even the most fit and athletic people. I, myself, do not perform enough flexibility training. While flexibility is slowly lost as we age, muscle-strengthening work also contributes to a loss of flexibility. If you engage in flexibility exercises alongside strength training, you will avoid the side effect of decreased range of motion, having the best of both worlds.

As we age, we become less flexible. This is due to certain changes that take place in our connective tissues. Our bodies gradually dehydrate as we age, causing decreased fluid within connective tissue fibers and more adhesions between these fibers. Stretching helps prevent the formation of such adhesions in the muscle and tendon fibers, combining nicely with the muscle and tendon breakdown and repair that come with strength training.

It becomes increasingly important to incorporate stretching exercises into your daily regimen as you age. Perhaps the best time to stretch is after your workout with weights or cardio, as the muscles have been warmed up. This also helps to keep adhesions from forming within the muscle and tendon tissues during the tissue recovery and repair time. Another good time to stretch is early in the morning, soon after waking. Think about it. What does a cat, a dog, or pretty much any mammal do immediately upon waking? They all stretch, and so should we!

When stretching, always remember to stretch to the point of resistance, not to the point of pain. Stretching too far could result in injury to the muscle or tendon that is under tension from the stretching exercise. Perform stretches for approximately ten minutes a day. Stretch each muscle group for at least a twenty-second hold before releasing. Stretch all muscles of the body that you can, but please make sure you stretch the hamstrings. This muscle stretches across both the hip and the knee joints and can greatly affect your gait when walking or running if tight. Tight hamstrings cause less range of motion in the hips and knees, have a negative effect on the lower back, and could lead to muscle tightness about the entire spinal axis. Loss of the normal range of motion in joints leads to degenerative changes. Less motion means less synovial fluid being released into the joints. (Synovial fluid is normally produced and released in response to the motion of a joint, protecting the joint from wearing away with constant motion.) With less synovial fluid, there is less joint lubrication and less delivery of nutrients to the joint tissues, leading to joint degeneration.

A good way to get your flexibility training in is to attend a yoga class or pop in a DVD and perform yoga sessions in your own home. Yoga is very effective not only for flexibility but for strength and balance as well. Yoga is also a great tool for relaxation; many people feel yoga helps with their stress levels more than any other exercise or activity.

There are several different types of yoga. I personally prefer Bikram yoga, as this form is practiced in a hundred-degree heated room for better flexibility of the muscles and tendons. It also causes you to sweat more during the workout, which is good for the release of toxins.

CARDIORESPIRATORY TRAINING

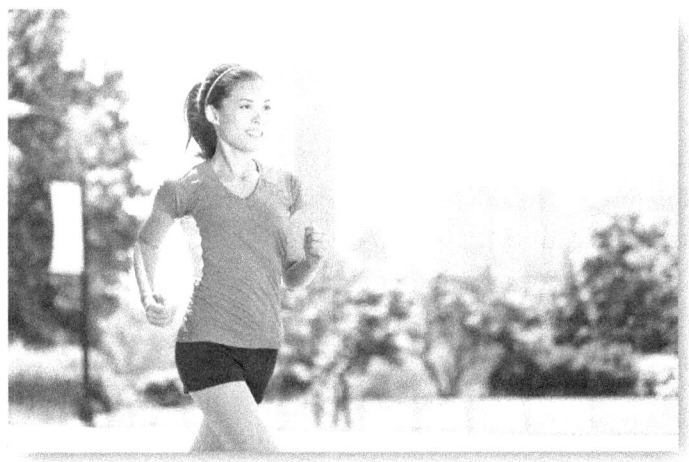

Cardiorespiratory training helps improve your heart and lung functions and also increases your sense of well-being. The term *cardiorespiratory* refers to the ability of the cardiovascular and respiratory systems to supply oxygen to skeletal muscles during a sustained bout of physical activity, such as a moderate jog, a bike ride, a swim, and so on. You can improve your cardiorespiratory function, or aerobic capacity, by performing any type of prolonged exercise that increases your aerobic energy system. Any exercise activity that increases your heart rate and keeps it elevated for a prolonged period is considered cardio exercise. Running, jogging, swimming, biking, brisk walking, and even sex are examples of activities that fit into this category.

When you exercise regularly, your body will become more efficient at supplying oxygen to muscle and other tissues. Your heart muscle will hypertrophy and become stronger, which will allow for more blood to be pumped with each beat. The number of small arteries in the exercised skeletal muscles will increase as a response to regular exercise, thereby supplying more blood to the working muscles. The respiratory system improves with exercise by increasing the amount of oxygen that is inhaled and distributed to the tissues.

Your body's ability to transport oxygen to your muscles and other tissues requires precise coordination between your heart, arteries, veins, and lungs. Oxygen transportation from the outside air to its eventual destination—your body's cells—happens this way:

1. Air is inhaled into the lungs.
2. The oxygen in the air is absorbed into the bloodstream via capillaries surrounding the lungs.
3. Then oxygen, attached now to the hemoglobin within the red blood cells, is transported via the pulmonary vein into the left atrium of the heart.
4. The oxygenated blood in the left atrium flows into the left ventricle as the valve between the atrium and ventricle opens.
5. The oxygenated blood is pumped out of the strong, muscular left ventricle of the heart and into the arteries that deliver it throughout the body—to muscles and other tissues.

6. When the oxygenated blood reaches the muscles, the oxygen is absorbed into the muscle cells from the capillaries that surround them.
7. While the blood is providing oxygen to the muscles, the blood is also removing carbon dioxide (CO_2, a waste product from cellular respiration) away from the tissues.
8. The deoxygenated blood, with the attached CO_2, is returned to the right atrium of the heart via the veins.
9. The right ventricle fills with the deoxygenated and CO_2-rich blood upon the opening of the right atrioventricular valve.
10. The right ventricle pumps blood out to the lungs.
11. The CO_2 is transferred from the blood to the lungs.
12. Once in the lungs, the CO_2 is released into the air through exhalation.
13. Inhalation then follows, taking more oxygen in from the air, and the entire process repeats.

So in essence, aerobic training improves the ability of your heart, arteries, veins, and lungs to work together in transporting oxygen to your tissues and exporting CO_2 away from your tissues. Regular aerobic exercise can reduce your risk of many health conditions and diseases, such as heart disease, lung cancer, type 2 diabetes, and stroke. It naturally helps to lower elevated levels of blood pressure, cholesterol, triglycerides, and blood sugar.

The American College of Sports Medicine recommends aerobic exercise three to five times per week, for thirty to sixty minutes per session, at a moderate intensity that maintains the heart rate at 65 to 85 percent of the maximum heart rate. An easy way to calculate your maximum heart rate is to subtract your age in years from the number 220. So, for instance, if you are thirty-five years old, 220 − 35 = 185. You can assume your maximum heart rate is approximately 185 beats per minute. Therefore, in order to follow the target heart-rate zone of 65 to 85 percent of your maximum heart rate, you would want to keep your heart rate in the 120 to 157 beats-per-minute range while performing an aerobic workout. In order to keep track of this during your workouts, you will need to wear a heart-rate or pulse-rate monitor while exercising.

Interval Training

When most of us think of cardiorespiratory exercise, we think of the typical mundane, hour-long bout of exercise on the treadmill, elliptical machine, or stair-stepper. However, unless you enjoy long-duration cardio or are training for a high-endurance event such as a marathon or a long-distance cycling race, you're probably not getting very psyched up for your next trip to the gym to go through the same old exhilaration-lacking routine.

Nevertheless, there is a solution to this monotony: high-intensity interval training, also referred to as HIIT. This type of training is a method of cardiorespiratory training where you perform the same amount of total workload that would be performed in a longer bout of steady-paced cardio exercise but in a much shorter time.

This type of training includes periods of high-intensity cardiorespiratory exercise, combined with lower-intensity recovery periods in succession. This type of training is meant to diminish the duration of your cardio workout and to burn more body fat than long-duration, steady-paced cardio. Another great benefit of HIIT is that it actually increases the body's metabolism over a twenty-four-hour span after workout, making it far more effective than the long-duration cardio. There is also significant evidence that interval training is more appropriate for preserving lean muscle tissue while simultaneously burning calories from body fat.

HIIT is considered to be a more advanced form of training compared to the more traditional cardio exercise due to the higher-intensity and continuous changeups within each training session. It has quickly become popular with everyone from the most elite athletes to general fitness enthusiasts. Although this type of training is considered advanced, it may easily be modified to fit beginners, provided that they have no preexisting heart or cardiovascular conditions that may not respond well to such a variable-changing routine.

Interval training may be applied to nearly any type of cardiorespiratory activity; the desired activity could be walking, jogging, swimming, biking, and so forth. For example, if one is relatively fit and regularly walks as part of his or her exercise routine, short periods (two to five minutes) of jogging may be incorporated into the walking. If the individual is less fit or this is too intense at first, simply walking more briskly for a few minutes may be added into the mix instead. One must allow for recovery with lower intensity, followed by a repeat of the higher-intensity walking. If an individual is well-conditioned, the inclusion of sprints into his or her daily jogging or treadmill exercise is sufficient.

The Benefits of HIIT
HIIT has several benefits over steady-paced cardiorespiratory training, including the following:

- more calories burned in less time
- improved cardiorespiratory endurance
- decreased muscle catabolism (the breakdown of tissue)
- higher degree of increased beta-oxidation (the breakdown of fatty acids in the body for use as energy) of adipose tissue (body fat) than with steady-paced cardiorespiratory training
- improvements in arterial elasticity
- reduced monotony when performing cardiorespiratory exercise

Interval Training for Fat Loss
There is clinical evidence suggesting that interval training is actually more effective at burning fat than lower-intensity cardio exercise. A group of researchers at the University of Guelph in Canada studied the incorporation of bursts of higher-intensity exercise into low- or

moderate-intensity exercise, and the impact it has on beta-oxidation of body fat.[xiv]

The study included eight women in their early twenties who cycled for ten sets of four minutes of intense, high-paced peddling, followed by two minutes of rest. Over a two-week period, they completed seven interval workouts. The researchers found that beta-oxidation of body fat among the interval-trained group increased 36 percent after performing HIIT versus another group of women of the same age group and conditioning level who trained with low- to moderate-intensity, steady-paced training only. Moreover, these improvements were consistent regardless of the fitness level of the subjects before undertaking the interval training.

Interval Training for Lean Muscle
Steady-paced distance or long-duration cardiorespiratory training (generally in excess of sixty minutes) may lead to muscular wasting, as the body depletes carbohydrate stores and turns to the utilization of protein stores (muscle tissue) for fuel.

Interval training discourages muscle catabolism, while encouraging muscle anabolism (the building up of tissue), especially when performing sprint training with short (fifteen- to thirty-second) rest intervals between each sprint, or when adding in two- to five-minute intervals of resistance to an individual's cardio to increase the intensity. This may be accomplished by raising the incline on the treadmill or increasing the resistance on the stationary bike or elliptical machine.

As you've probably noticed when watching the Olympics, distance runners have very little muscle mass, while sprinters, on the other hand, tend to carry significantly more muscle mass (particularly in the quadriceps and hamstrings), while still maintaining extremely low body-fat levels. Sprinters typically train for short bursts of power and regularly utilize HIIT. One of the most effective methods of interval training is to substitute sprints for steady-paced cardio exercise.

Sprints can be performed as part of a street-running or jogging routine, on a treadmill at the gym, or at a local track. The most preferable type of area for performing sprints is at a track. The approach here is simple but highly effective: run or walk at a moderate pace for two to three minutes and then sprint at full speed for one minute. Return to the moderate pace for two to three minutes and continue repeating the cycle for up to thirty minutes total. Alternately, one may perform a full-speed sprint for fifty meters, rest for fifteen to thirty seconds, and repeat, for fifteen sprints total. The latter example would be for a well-conditioned, seasoned athlete or fitness enthusiast.

Keep in mind that the goal is not volume but intensity. Initially, you should not expect to be able to perform this more than a few times before feeling significant fatigue and soreness. Over time, the number of sprints in the training session can be raised to ten to fifteen, with fifteen to thirty seconds of rest in between sprints.

Including HIIT into Your Regimen
This type of training helps to alleviate the problem of boredom that is so commonly associated with duration cardio training. It is the new wave in fitness today and rightfully so. With increasing clinical evidence of its superiority over duration cardio training for fat loss as well as decreased catabolism of muscle tissue, this type of training is appealing to athletes and fitness enthusiasts of all levels.

Train Hard, Train Regularly, but Don't Overtrain

With the main point of this chapter being how to increase your activity and live a more active lifestyle, it is important to also note there are limits for us all in reference to frequency of exercise and recovery time from each exercise bout.

For the average person who exercises regularly, overtraining generally isn't a problem, as most will struggle just to maintain regular workout sessions around their busy lives. However, there are some people who may be somewhat addicted to training, sometimes even going so far as multiple workout sessions per day with inadequate recovery in between.

Although a select few can handle multiple sessions per day on a daily basis (this would only be for the sponsored athletes, whose job it is to train and compete, and therefore have time to rest between the bouts), most people have careers that are not in the sports realm, attend school, or have a family to care for. So multiple workouts per day would be unfeasible for them.

Most people who train regularly want to get into better shape, lose a few pounds, and have a healthier life. Often when people see great results from their training, it is natural for them to feel like more would be better. The fact that recovery is where the actual growth in muscle mass and increase in myofibrils take place is far too often not understood by those who train.

If you reduce the amount of rest and recovery, the body cannot make itself stronger. It's like continuously scraping the scab off a wound, not allowing it time to heal before inflicting stress onto the area again. If you engage in another bout of intense training before enough time for proper recovery has elapsed, you are undoubtedly overtraining.

After the onset of high-intensity training exercise, a hormone known as cortisol is released from the adrenal cortex, which breaks down proteins into their constituent amino acids and sends them to the liver for conversion to glucose. The longer the workout, the more cortisol is pumped in, and the more protein is destroyed. This causes a "catabolic state," because the largest supply of protein lies in the muscles, so cortisol will act on the breakdown there primarily.

Overtraining results in several unwanted consequences, such as a weakened immune system, increased susceptibility to injuries, persistent delayed-onset muscle soreness, fatigue, irritability, depression, insomnia, loss of appetite, and loss of motivation.

Overtraining can force the body into a weakened physical state, which could produce a cold or the flu, or worse, could tear muscles, tendons, and ligaments once those tissues lose their structural integrity due to protein loss from the increased levels of cortisol. The increased likelihood of illness is due to the fact that the immune system is based on proteins, and the influx of cortisol into the bloodstream takes up the proteins that are normally used to make up the immune system, such as white blood cells and other constituents.

To avoid this overtraining quandary, careful planning for one's training regimen must be undertaken. Several important aspects of one's training program should be closely examined, such as the timing of the higher-intensity sessions in relation to those of low-intensity, making sufficient time for rest and recovery between workout sessions, and proper nutrition for the trainee's optimal recovery.

One must also look at the daily activities that are involved in his or her life as far as career and hobbies are concerned, as too much stress will greatly affect his or her recovery from intense training sessions.

It is important to emphasize carbohydrate intake. Around 60 to 70 percent of the total caloric intake is optimal for recovery purposes. Carbohydrates should be consumed two hours prior to exercising and immediately following exercise. Research has shown that your fatigued muscles appear to be most responsive to energy storage (the energy storage of kilocalories, specifically glucose) within the first thirty minutes following your workout. There is a lesser response for the next ten hours.

Protein intake is also a very important factor. Protein should be consumed one to two hours before and immediately following exercise. Research has shown that the body is also more receptive to protein immediately following a workout.

Post-exercise muscle glycogen storage can be enhanced with a combination carbohydrate-protein supplement as a result of the interaction of carbohydrates and protein on insulin secretion. The addition of protein with carbohydrates will allow for a more rapid recovery. Drink a rehydration beverage during and after exercise to quickly replace electrolytes as well as glucose.

One more factor, and this one is the most crucial: adequate water must be consumed. The body functions optimally when it is fully hydrated. It is recommended for an athlete or an individual who engages in any type of moderate to intense training to consume at least 128 ounces (one gallon) of water daily. During the warm summer months, it may be most appropriate to double this amount in order to ensure proper hydration.

CHAPTER 3

LOOKING YOUNGER

ONE OF THE main reasons you picked up this book in the first place was probably that the idea of looking younger is very enticing. We all want to look and feel younger. As we have gone over the dietary aspects of how you may slow aging with the right nutrition, we also need to focus on your skin.

Your skin is forced to face many harmful factors as you age: ultraviolet (UV) radiation from the sun, harsh weather and climate changes, air pollution, cigarette smoking or secondhand smoke, and so on. Some of this is within our control, but much of it is not. We can take certain measures to protect our skin in order to have the supple and radiant look that we all desire.

First of all, good diet and loading up on antioxidants are just as important for protecting the nature of your skin. In practically every aspect of slowing down the aging process, diet is king. With that being said, there are other steps to take involving Botox, microderm abrasion, other medical skin treatments, topical skin care products, and nutrition taken internally and externally.

BEST FOODS FOR HEALTHY SKIN AND HAIR

First, look to your diet when considering actions for preventing or decreasing lines and wrinkles. Nothing works better than properly nourishing your skin, hair, and nails from within. You can apply the greatest, most expensive lotion on the market all day long, every day, yet not receive even close to the optimal results of skin nourishment that you would get from having a diet that is rich in antioxidants, certain minerals and vitamins, proteins, and essential fatty acids.

Let's look at some of the best foods for your skin, hair, and nails. You should eat a wide variety of these foods to get the best results, being that each has its own unique density of certain nutrients.

Blueberries

You can't go wrong adding blueberries to any meal. These berries are jam-packed with antioxidant-rich, free-radical-fighting nutrients that deliver many health benefits, including better skin. The blueberry was ranked number one in antioxidant activity by the US Department of Agriculture, compared to forty common fruits and vegetables, as mentioned in a *Fitness* magazine article written by nutritionist Lisa Drayer (author of *The Beauty Diet*).[xv] The antioxidants in blueberries may protect your skin from premature aging, so you should add half a cup to your protein smoothie, yogurt, or porridge daily.

Acai Berries

There are many skin products on the market today containing acai oil due to the antioxidant-rich nature of the oil. This oil is quite moisturizing and nourishing for your skin and is a natural alternative to many other chemical skin products. Nevertheless, the nutrients from this berry, as in any other food, are best utilized internally. So whether you are using this oil on your skin, remember to place the berries in your diet first and foremost.

Wild-Caught Salmon

Wild salmon, meaning not farm raised, is a prime choice for omega-3 fatty acids, which help keep your skin supple and moisturized. Salmon also contains the mineral selenium, which helps in protecting your skin from sun exposure. Salmon is also a good source of vitamin D, which works with calcium and other nutrients to make your bones and teeth strong and healthy. Wild-caught salmon is truly a superfood that should be a staple in your diet.

OYSTERS

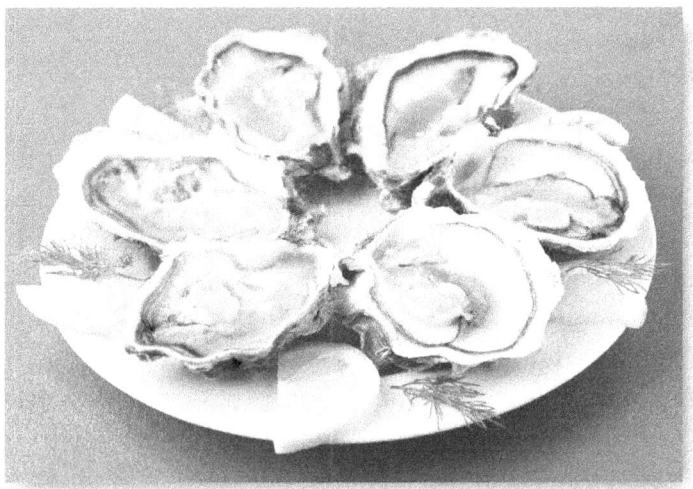

Oysters are a great food choice for your skin, hair, and nails because of the high content of zinc found in these mollusks. Zinc has a role in skin-cell renewal and repair and in supporting a healthy, robust structure in the hair and nails.

WALNUTS

Walnuts, the healthiest of all in the nutritious food family of nuts and seeds, are another food high in omega-3 fatty acids, which bestow the age-defying benefits of healthier skin, hair, and nails, not to mention omega-3s' benefits to the heart, eyes, and bones. You can easily obtain an entire daily dose of omega-3s and vitamin E from just a small handful of walnuts. You can simply add this, along with your blueberries, to your daily porridge or yogurt every morning to start your day off in the right direction.

KIWIFRUIT

Kiwifruit is another fruit loaded with vitamin C and antioxidants. Vitamin C is an important nutrient for the health of collagen in your skin. Healthy, robust collagen fibers allow for firm skin, thereby helping to prevent wrinkles. Many of the antioxidants in a kiwifruit may help prevent cardiovascular diseases and cancer.

KALE

I dare say that the single most important food you should include in your diet is kale. In the past, when I would have people come up to me and ask, "What can I do if I want to lose a whole bunch of weight in just a couple weeks and not hurt myself in the process?" I would say, "Kale and water." Now, obviously we need much more than that, but this food is loaded with antioxidant vitamins and minerals, high in fiber, has extremely low-calorie content, and has high omega-3s; no single food can really match it.

With such high-antioxidant content, kale is also a prime choice for anti-aging purposes. Your skin requires a healthy dose of vitamin A, one of the many nutrients for which kale is a good source. Vitamin A is necessary in repairing the tissues underneath your skin and helps prevent damage caused by free radicals. Without sufficient amounts of vitamin A, your skin will become dry and flaky.

This leaf also contains a high amount of vitamin K, which supports your skin's elasticity. Vitamin C is very prevalent in kale, therefore helping to reduce free-radical damage and to support the skin by adding collagen content. Kale even contains omega-3 and omega-6 fatty acids, which aid in the health of the skin and hair in many ways.

These foods are some of the most important ones to include in your diet for healthy, radiant skin. For better skin, hair, and nails, you should strive to eat more foods that are high in omega-3 fatty acids; vitamins A, C, and K; and zinc.

WORST FOODS FOR HEALTHY SKIN AND HAIR

Now we will uncover some of the worst foods for your skin. There are foods out there that invite rashes, blemishes, and breakouts. Beware of these, or they will prove detrimental to your outer shell. These foods need to be eliminated from your diet as much as possible, if you want smooth, supple skin with a nice complexion.

AVOID SUGARY FOODS

According to dermatologist Valori Treloar (author of *The Clear Skin*), blood sugar plays a role in skin health. Foods that spike your insulin level will lead to acne and breakouts. Treloar explained to WebMD that a good way to improve your skin health is to eat in a manner that keeps your blood sugar steady. Some foods will cause your blood sugar level to rise quickly, triggering your body to secrete a large amount of insulin into the bloodstream to help your body's cells absorb the excessive amount of sugar present in the blood.

According to Treloar, "[when you're] eating a cookie, you're eating a granola bar, and you're drinking a sweetened beverage, you're pushing your blood sugar up high and fast, and you're going to have more insulin circulating in your bloodstream."

According to Eric Metcalf of WebMD, a 2007 research study supports a positive link between higher blood sugar levels and the presence of skin acne. The study ran for three months, included forty-three teenage boys and young men with acne, and separated the subjects into two classifications: some ate low-glycemic foods, while others consumed foods with a high-glycemic load. The study found that those who consumed the prescribed low-glycemic diet had more improvement in their acne.

DON'T HAVE TOO MUCH DAIRY

The jury is still out on any links between dairy and acne. However, there is some credible research demonstrating such a connection. A 2008 article in the *Journal of the American Academy of Dermatology* suggested that dairy consumption may be a cause of acne.[xvi] Milk contains components related to the hormone testosterone. This hormone will stimulate oil glands in the skin, thereby contributing to acne outbreaks. So, if dairy has an impact on the rise of testosterone production and/or release into the bloodstream, this would justify such a connection between dairy consumption and skin acne.

BALANCE OUT YOUR FATS

Fats in our food can worsen or lower inflammation in the body, depending on which types of fatty acids are consumed. High inflammation present in your body can show up on your skin. Before the dawn of processed foods and the methods we use to cook and prepare meals now, omega-3 and omega-6 fatty acids were nearly at a one-to-one ratio in people's diets. Unfortunately, omega-6s are much more prevalent in people's diets now, creating an imbalance between the two.

A simple solution would be to use less vegetable oils such as corn, safflower, and canola oil, as all of these have higher levels of omega-6s. Also, the animal foods you consume, such as poultry, eggs, and beef, should be free range or from roaming pastures, instead of non-roaming and corn fed. Finally, you should eat more fish (such as salmon) that is high in omega-3s, and take fish oil supplements.

EFFECTIVE SKIN TREATMENTS FOR ANTI-AGING

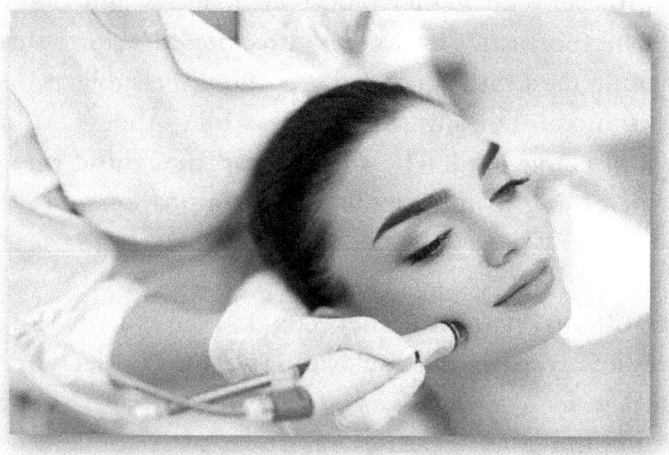

BOTOX

The popularity of Botox has risen considerably, particularly with people in their twenties and thirties, as dermatologists and plastic surgeons commonly suggest beginning this treatment before wrinkles begin to naturally show. There is good reason for this suggestion, given what a wrinkle actually is from an anatomical standpoint.

Julius W. Few, an assistant professor of plastic surgery at Northwestern University's Feinberg School of Medicine in Chicago, explains it this way in an interview with WebMD on the topic of the Botox trend among younger people:

> As one gets older and loses some of the elasticity of the skin, creases and wrinkles become more permanent...[I]t's not unreasonable to believe that doing some preventive things now such as using sunscreen or getting Botox injections may stave off the process...It is a reasonable kind of impression that if someone were to have maintenance Botox injections fairly regularly then theoretically they may be able to slow the development of wrinkles...And for people in their late 20s or early 30s who have just the beginning of creases or depressions in their frown line, Botox is a great option because it can eliminate these problems and may also be able to slow the development of a deeper crease.[xvii]

However, Few does go on to note that wrinkle prevention from Botox treatment has yet to be scientifically proven.

Botox injections work by blocking signals known as neurotransmitters from the nerve fiber's synapse with a muscle fiber, essentially decreasing the ability of the muscle fiber to contract. So, for a facial muscle that is injected with Botox, it can no longer contract, causing the wrinkles to relax and soften.

Botox treatments generally keep the muscles injected in a relaxed state for four to six months, which is why physicians will accordingly suggest follow-up treatments after that same length of time. The cost for a Botox procedure usually ranges from $350 to $600. Men typically require more Botox than women, due to the greater muscle mass in men.

DYSPORT

Dysport is a relatively new treatment to the United States and one that people are finding to be a good alternative to Botox. It was developed in the early 1990s in the United Kingdom and then was approved by the US Food and Drug Administration in 2009 for the treatment of head and neck muscle spasms and for cosmetic purposes.

Dysport is very similar to Botox in that both work the same way. It is made from the same botulinum toxin (type A) as Botox and is injected in the same way as well. From a chemical standpoint, there is a slight difference in the makeup in that Dysport has fewer proteins surrounding the toxin than in the case of Botox. For this reason, the toxin in Dysport may stimulate a weaker immune response for the body to break down the toxin in comparison to Botox. This may make it a good option for Botox patients who feel that Botox no longer works because their bodies have developed antibodies. There are some claims to support that Dysport works faster and lasts longer than Botox. It is also slightly cheaper than Botox in most clinics and medical spas.

MICRODERM ABRASION

Microderm abrasion is one of the more recent skin care techniques that are trendy now. Many satisfied customers describe it as an "instant face-lift." This is indeed an effective alternative to plastic surgery, chemical peels, and Botox injections.

Microderm abrasion is a procedure for the skin that involves the application of tiny rough grains to buff away the surface layer of skin. Many different products and treatments use this method, including medical procedures, salon treatments, and exfoliating scrubs that you apply yourself at home. This treatment is typically performed on the face, chest, neck, arms, or hands—areas where skin is most often exposed. To understand how this treatment works, it is important to comprehend some of the general anatomy of the skin.

Your skin is comprised of two main layers—the inner layer, known as the dermis, and the outer layer, known as the epidermis. Epidermis actually has five layers, one layer on top of another. The lower layers of the epidermis consist of cells in the process of maturing. As the outermost layer at the top of the skin (called the stratum corneum) is sloughed off, the younger epidermal cells are exposed.

It is this top layer of the skin that microderm abrasion sloughs off, exposing the next maturest level of epidermal cells underneath. The theory behind this method is that by removing the older, dead cells of the stratum corneum, the body sees this as a mild injury. This would elicit a response that would speed up the natural process of regenerating new, healthier skin cells to replace those that have been lost.

There are several different types of microderm abrasion. For instance, in the commercial version that you would see in a medical spa, a specialized instrument would be applied by a dermatologist or trained technician. This instrument works by shooting a stream of microcrystals of aluminum oxide, sodium chloride, or sodium bicarbonate onto the surface of the skin to instantly wear away the outermost skin cells. Other types of microderm abrasion include home treatments using scrubs and creams that contain the same microcrystals, though professional treatment in a clinic is recommended for best results.

The traditional crystal-based microderm abrasion system includes a vacuum mechanism, which has four basic roles: (1) it gently pulls the skin, lifting it for abrasion; (2) it sprays a stream of crystals across the area of lifted skin; (3) it stimulates blood circulation in the treated area; and (4) it collects the dead skin and used crystals for disposal.

Your skin typically regenerates in thirty-day intervals, so most clinicians recommend this treatment every two to four weeks. Usually six to twelve treatments are needed in order see a significant improvement in your skin.

The healing process resulting from this procedure allows for newer skin cells at the top skin layer, which look and feel smoother. This treatment is an effective and economical way to remove sun damage, blemishes, and fine lines on your skin. Skin creams and lotions are more effective if you regularly have this treatment because more of the active ingredients may penetrate deeper into the lower layers of skin.

Professional treatments that you would get from a dermatologist or medical spa would cost around $100 to $200 per session, typically with several sessions spaced throughout the year for maximum effectiveness. Home treatments such as microderm abrasion creams and scrubs are typically priced in the range of $50 to $80 per jar.

CHEMICAL SKIN PEEL

Chemical skin peel is not a new concept at all. It is one of the oldest cosmetic procedures in the world, as it was performed in ancient Egypt, Greece, and Rome on people who wanted to have smoother, better-looking skin. Chemical facial peels are very popular now because of the nearly immediate results from the procedure.

With a chemical peel, an acid solution is used to remove the damaged outer layers of the skin. The acid solution of alpha-hydroxy acids, trichloroacetic acid, or phenol is applied to the skin by a physician.

Typically administered as a facial peel, a chemical peel enhances the texture of the skin. It is an effective treatment for facial blemishes, wrinkles, and uneven skin pigmentation. Similar in principle to microderm abrasion, this type of treatment also works by exfoliating the outer layers of dead skin, exposing a younger skin layer that has better texture and tone. Chemical skin peels may be full facials or spot treatments for mild skin disfigurements such as stretch marks or unsightly scars. More invasive, yet perhaps more effective, are deep chemical peels. This type of peel involves a longer procedure with a recovery time of between two to six months. Patients who want to correct skin disfigurements or discolorations brought on by sun exposure, or lessen unsightly wrinkles, may benefit from a deep chemical peel. This treatment may be more than an hour long and may require sedation. If you go with a deep peel, expect a long, slow recovery period, and please remember to wear sunscreen whenever you are out in the sun.

The cost of a full-facial chemical skin peel is usually between $600 and $1,000. Deep chemical peels are priced as high as $6,000.

PLATELET-RICH PLASMA (PRP) SKIN REGENERATION

PRP is a new and increasingly popular technique in the clinical world of anti-aging treatments. This form of treatment is popular in physical medicine, as it has the potential benefits of aiding in wound healing, recovery from tendinitis, and healing from various surgical procedures (and other soft-tissue injuries). Regarding its place in cosmetic treatment, PRP can potentially help reverse the common signs of aging in the skin, specifically in the areas of the face, neck, and hands. The advantage of PRP over other common anti-aging treatments such as Botox is its natural quality. The therapy uses the patient's own blood, making the treatment hypoallergenic.

PRP skin rejuvenation therapy uses components of the blood known as platelets. Platelets play a role in stopping bleeding and repairing damaged blood vessels and cells in the body. Platelets contain molecular substances known as growth factors, which activate and rejuvenate cells. The growth factors, when released, induce the production of collagen and the generation of new capillaries to rejuvenate the skin.

The most common conditions treated with PRP skin rejuvenation therapy include fine wrinkles around the eyes, nasolabial grooves, wrinkles on or around the lips, acne marks, wrinkles on the forehead, wrinkles on the neck, bags and dark circles under the eyes, loose and saggy skin, and scars.

For separation of PRP in the blood, a specific filter and centrifuge is used by the physician to achieve a high platelet-recovery rate (usually 95 percent or more), allowing the preparation of plasma containing six to ten times as many platelets (density-wise) as normal blood plasma.

The steps for PRP therapy are as follows. First, the blood is collected from the patient. Next, a specialized filter and centrifuge are used to prepare PRP, containing autologous white blood cells. Finally, this PRP with autologous white blood cells is injected into the area targeted for treatment. The entire process is completed in one office visit, taking about thirty to forty minutes from blood collection to injection of the PRP.

Platelets and white blood cells exert a synergistic effect on the treated areas, resulting in the release of growth factors at the injection sites. This promotes the production of collagen and hyaluronic acid, which helps wound healing and improves skin imperfections such as wrinkles, acne marks, scars, and loose skin via dermal or soft-tissue regeneration.

PRP skin rejuvenation therapy may provide benefits for loose skin under the eyes, which is difficult to treat with conventional rejuvenating injections and laser therapy. Because PRP therapy uses the patient's own blood for rejuvenation, any risk of infection or allergy is practically nil. It has the advantage of a longer duration of efficacy compared with the injection of hyaluronic acid and collagen that are absorbed into the body. There is also no need for skin incision. Patients have a short downtime with this type of therapy, as swelling usually resolves in two to three hours.

Overall, PRP therapy for skin rejuvenation is a very safe treatment. The effectiveness is still up for debate among researchers and practitioners, as limited research has been spent covering the effectiveness of this therapy in the realms of either soft-tissue healing or cosmetic treatments. However, many case studies have illustrated PRP therapy's success both in physical medicine and in skin rejuvenation; the evidence certainly appears to be growing, from my personal experience with patients in my clinics, and from that of my colleagues around the world.

LASER SKIN RESURFACING

If you choose to look at slightly more invasive procedures, laser skin resurfacing has proven very effective as line and wrinkle reduction or removal.

This treatment diminishes the appearance of imperfections on the surface of the skin. It helps reduce the effects of the sun, aging, and certain facial-skin disorders. During the procedure, a laser is used to dissolve the molecular bonds of the damaged skin cells, layer by layer, until a smoother and clearer skin appearance is achieved.

The procedure has similar anti-aging benefits as microderm abrasion or chemical skin peels, as this, too, works on tearing down or removing the outer skin layer, although laser skin resurfacing does take this to another level. The laser penetrates deeper into the epidermis, removing multiple epidermal layers of damaged skin cells, hence rejuvenating the skin.

Laser skin resurfacing is generally performed by a dermatologist or plastic surgeon and usually costs around $2,200 to $3,000 in most cities.

FACELIFT

Having a facelift is the most expensive treatment option if you're looking to remove fine lines and wrinkles. Going to this extreme does have outstanding results in many cases. This procedure became very popular in the 1980s, yet there were many ho-hum results in its earlier stages, as the surgery was focused purely on tightening the skin, not paying attention to the underlying facial muscles and fat beneath the skin. The results from these early facelifts usually looked rather artificial, instead of youthful. Now when you have a facelift procedure, your plastic surgeon will not only remove the excess skin but will also tighten the facial muscles and remove excess fat. Facelift surgery usually addresses the neck, chin, lower part of the face, and around the nose.

Having a facelift is not cheap—ranging anywhere from $3,000 to $15,000, depending on how much of the face is worked on, which city the procedure is performed in, and who is the surgeon.

SKIN LOTIONS AND OILS

There is a consistently rising number of skin care topicals on the market today, a reflection on our society's fear of growing old. Many of these products claim some amazing benefits to their use; however, the evidence to back up such claims is lacking in most instances. In an interview with WebMD, dermatologist and New York University professor Rhanda Narins noted, "Many of these products are claiming changes in the skin that would automatically classify them as drugs, and they are not." There is a largely misleading message these skin care–product companies are putting out to the public, no doubt.

Still, there are benefits to the use of some skin creams, lotions, and oils that should be addressed. To better separate the helpful skin topicals from the hundreds of useless ones out there, it is important that you know the ingredients the products contain as well as those ingredients' benefits. To better understand which creams and lotions can actually make an impact on skin health and anti-aging practices, let's look further into some of the molecular makeup of the skin.

The look of aging skin is primarily due to the loss of collagen. Collagen is a connective tissue substance that, in your skin's dermis layer, is mostly responsible for strength and pliability, keeping your skin from forming lines and wrinkles. We naturally lose collagen fibers in the skin and in most other connective tissues slowly as we age; however, environmental factors such as lack of proper nutrition, sun exposure, smoking, and pollution will further encourage collagen loss. These environmental factors, as well as the natural aging process of our cells, result in the release of free radicals that destroy collagen fibers.

Returning to the discussion on the wonderful antioxidants in certain foods, we also have antioxidants in skin creams that may be of benefit in disabling free radicals before they destroy the collagen in the skin. There is little evidence to support such products' ability to effectively protect the skin, but in theory, it wouldn't hurt to give your skin that added support. Just keep in mind that diet is king; nothing beats a healthy diet rich in a wide range of antioxidants.

Furthermore, many skin lotions and creams have some degree of sunscreen, which have the obvious benefit of limiting sun exposure and skin damage. You must look closely at each product's description to know whether it has such protection (SPF). Note also that it is recommended by most dermatologists to have at least an SPF of 15 or higher (30 or higher if one has fair skin) if one is in the sun for more than fifteen minutes. Aside from sunscreen lotions, most lotions and creams do not have a high SPF rating.

USE SUNSCREEN

At the beach, one often sees at least one person out there with skin the color of a lobster. Sunscreen is easy to apply, not that expensive, and can save us from lots of discomfort from sunburns, not to mention long-term damage to the skin. Yet so often, we are reluctant to apply it when we go out in the sun for an extended period.

There are two different ways sunscreens can shield the skin from the dangerous ultraviolet (UV) rays. Some sunscreens cause the UV light to scatter when it hits the body where the sunscreen was applied, effectively reflecting the UV light away from the skin. Other types work by absorbing the UV rays before they reach the skin.

Sunscreens used to protect our skin from only UVB light, which is the type that actually causes our skin to burn. Today, many sunscreens protect against both UVA and UVB. This is due to research studies revealing that UVA light also increases skin cancer, perhaps just as much as UVB rays, even though UVA rays are not a cause for sunburn. UVA rays are also just as apt to penetrate deeply and cause damage that will bring about wrinkles. According to an article at WebMD, the Environmental Protection Agency estimates that up to 90 percent of skin changes associated with aging are caused by a lifetime of exposure to UVA rays.[xviii] Therefore, UVA rays are at least as damaging as UVB rays.

SPF is a rating that refers to only UVB blockage. There is no rating in place for the protection that sunscreens have against UVA rays. So it is important that you pay close attention to the ingredients in the product. When shopping, you will need to first look for a sunscreen with broad-spectrum or multispectrum protection for both UVB and UVA. In an interview with WebMD, David J. Leffell, professor of dermatology and surgery at the Yale School of Medicine, said we should look for these UVA-blocking ingredients: ecamsule, avobenzone, oxybenzone, titanium dioxide, sulisobenzone, or zinc oxide.

If you are going to be in the water or are planning on exercising while out in the sunlight, be sure to use a water- and sweat-resistant sunscreen lotion. You will also need to reapply every hour; otherwise, the sunscreen will lose its protective quality.

CHAPTER 4

HORMONE REPLACEMENT THERAPY (FEEL LIKE YOU'RE TWENTY-FIVE AGAIN)

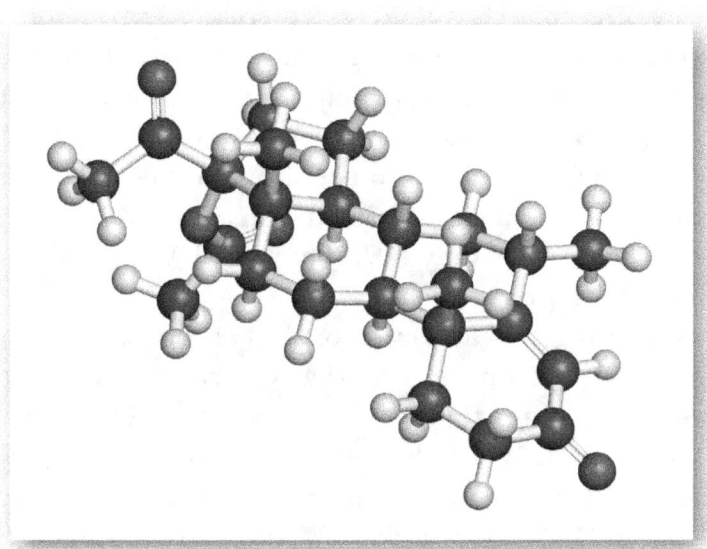

YOUR BODY'S HORMONE production will change as you age. The stress in your life will impact your physical, mental, and emotional well-being. Stress and the aging of your body's organs will alter the demands on your hormonal system and the ability of your body to adequately produce and release certain hormones. These hormones are necessary for living a healthier, more vivacious life.

Imbalances in natural production of hormones affect both men and women. In recent years, we have been fortunate to have therapies available to us that may decrease the effects of aging and slow the aging process.

With such therapies that help create a better balance within your hormones, you will experience more energy throughout the day, better sleep at night, increased sex drive, better mental focus and alertness, and a better sense of well-being. Feeling young again is now more of a reality than ever for middle-aged folks who want to feel like they did in their twenties again.

If you are in your thirties or older, and you have symptoms of insomnia, irritability, fatigue, lack of energy or pep, decreased libido, skin dryness, vaginal dryness if you're female, erectile dysfunction if you're male, or memory loss, you could be dealing with a hormonal imbalance. Having a hormone imbalance can cause a weakened immune system, an increase in blood sugar levels, a loss of bone density, more likelihood of muscle or tendon strains or tears, changes in blood pressure, and more. With your hormones out of sync, your body wears down, and you just don't have a healthy sense of well-being.

Hormone Replacement for Women

For a woman, aging is difficult enough, but the declining levels of hormones make things all the more difficult. With such a drop in these levels, you will suffer from a diminished sense of well-being, have less energy, and lose your libido, among a list of other symptoms. The good news is that you don't have to accept this passively. You can restore your hormone levels with hormone replacement therapy (HRT) and allow yourself the feeling of being in your twenties or early thirties again.

I cannot stress enough the importance of proper hormone balance. This truly is the fountain of youth in many ways, especially for women. Once you begin your treatment, it may take a few trials and errors as your doctor finds the proper balance for you individually. However, when you do find the right balance, you will be glad you chose to take action with your hormones.

There are different types of HRT out there. I would like to focus primarily on bioidentical hormone replacement therapy (BHRT), as this is the safer alternative, with the least amount of side effects. The reason is that the body basically eliminates any excess amounts of a bioidentical hormone in the body, keeping your levels from being too high for your body to handle properly. Synthetic hormone medications, on the other hand, could grow to unnatural and unsafe levels in the body, if not carefully watched, leading to unwanted side effects such as restlessness, anxiety, diminished mental focus, acne and other skin problems, among others. While the jury is still out as to whether BHRT is truly safer than synthetic, there are studies demonstrating the safety in regard to BHRT over synthetic, in men and women alike. Currently, the US Food and Drug Administration does not have enough evidence to justify that bioidentical hormones are safer or more effective than other hormone products, and therefore currently suggests that the benefits and risks are likely to be the same with BHRT or synthetic HRT. To put it simply, there are not enough studies to clearly and conclusively state that BHRT is safer than HRT in either sex. However, it is worth knowing how these chemicals break down in your body and the evidence that points to BHRT being the safer option in both sexes.

Combining hormone replacement with proper diet and an active lifestyle will allow you to feel like you did in your twenties, boosting your energy as well as improving your outlook on life, and could very well help you return to the best shape of your life. When it comes to maximizing your living years for general enjoyment of life, staying healthy and fit is the only tried-and-true method. Balancing your hormones will put you in the right direction, making you feel much better overall. And when you feel better and have a healthier outlook on life, you are more likely to adopt other lifestyle changes such as improved diet and exercise, which all work synergistically to reinforce an improved sense of well-being.

Many women tend to go untreated for their symptoms from menopause. Hot flashes, mood swings, irritability, poor mental focus, and difficulty in falling or staying asleep at night are all signs of estrogen deficiency. Women with estrogen deficiency usually have more difficulty in concentration and cannot focus on a particular task at hand in the way they could when they were younger, when hormone levels were healthier. Commonly, energy levels are diminished to the point of being classified as chronic fatigue in women with dwindling estrogen levels. This deficiency also produces feelings of depression and a decreased sense of self-worth.

When you bring these compounding symptoms together, you can expect a lack of exercise, less-than-stellar eating habits, and weight gain. You will also have a lack of sex drive with hormone imbalance. The snowballing effect can go on and on, making hormone imbalance a tougher hill to climb the longer you go without tackling the problem.

The symptoms of hormone imbalance are a result of hormone deficiency—they are not actually attributable to the normal aging process. We all see a drop in hormone levels as we age, but aging itself is not to blame. While you cannot reverse the aging process, you can certainly optimize your physical health, well-being, and vigor by restoring the normal balance of estrogen, progesterone, and testosterone that has been negatively affected by menopause. When you restore your body's normal balance of hormones, you will quickly begin to feel younger, healthier, and happier. You will live with more vivacity—the way your life is meant to be lived.

HRT and BHT can help balance your hormones and improve your health. Whether you are a candidate for HRT and whether you should go with the bioidentical or synthetic route are questions that should be discussed with your doctor. After all, everyone has different needs based on a superfluity of components. You will need a treatment plan that is designed uniquely for you and one that you can follow in order to successfully get your hormones at the right levels.

Keep in mind that you will maximize your results from HRT with a high-antioxidant, nutritious diet and regular exercise. Properly balanced hormones, diet, and exercise all work together. These are like pieces to a puzzle. They all have to be there, or the picture isn't all that great.

Hormone Replacement for Men

Many people regard HRT as a concern for only women. This is far from the truth. Men's testosterone levels peak in their late teens, and when men are about thirty years old, testosterone levels begin a gradual, steady decline of about 1 percent a year from then on, according to a 2012 study by the Mayo Clinic.[xix] If you are a man, aging comes with diminished levels of testosterone, just as women must deal with decreasing levels of estrogen and progesterone. Sometimes, women also deal with exceedingly diminished levels of testosterone themselves, as they also require some amount of testosterone. For women, all testosterone is produced in the adrenal glands. For men, testosterone comes predominantly from the testicles, specifically the leydig cells of the testicles. The adrenal glands are responsible for a smaller portion of testosterone release in men. Men who have decreased levels of testosterone are at increased risk for metabolic syndrome—a cluster of risk factors that include elevated cholesterol, high blood pressure, and an increased risk of heart disease, stroke, and type 2 diabetes, among other health conditions.

Testosterone is vital to a man for several reasons. Adequate blood levels of this hormone help maintain his bone density, muscle strength and mass, fat distribution, red blood cell production, facial and body hair, sex drive, and sperm production. Inadequate levels of testosterone may lead to decreased interest in sex, inability to have or keep an erection, insomnia, lethargy, depression, difficulty with concentration and memory, increased body fat, reduced muscle bulk and strength, and decreased bone density.

The goal of testosterone treatment, just as any other type of HRT, is to bring the body's levels into normal range. Low testosterone levels in men are obviously more common with increasing age, but males can have lower levels than the norm at any age. Women may also have lower testosterone levels than normal.

But while HRT has been linked to heart disease and other conditions in women, this doesn't appear to be the case with men. At this time, there is no substantiated increased risk of heart disease for men undergoing testosterone replacement therapy. Fundamentally, testosterone replacement in men is quite different from hormone replacement in women and has less risk.

In several studies, testosterone replacement therapy has been found to help testosterone-deficient men over forty to reduce their risk of heart disease, stroke, and diabetes. When properly managed, testosterone treatment helps to lower high blood pressure, lower LDLs (bad cholesterol), and raise HDLs (good cholesterol). In a recent study, within three months of testosterone treatment in men of widely ranging ages (ninety-five total subjects, from thirty-four to sixty-nine years of age), the subjects had lower cholesterol and triglycerides, as well as lower body mass index. Most men in the study lost their potbellies, losing about three to four inches off the waist in twelve months of therapy, and also reduced their total cholesterol by one-fourth to one-third after one year in the treatment.[xx]

The main caution regarding testosterone therapy is the increased risk of prostate cancer. It is widely known that cancer of the prostate is usually dependent on testosterone. Cancer in the prostate is usually a slow-growing tumor, and the presence of high levels of testosterone will encourage the tumor to grow faster. For this reason, it is strongly advised that men should have their prostates examined for cancer prior to beginning testosterone treatment. Men on testosterone therapy should also have routine prostate checkups throughout the duration of treatment.

Higher levels of testosterone also cause an increase in red blood cell count, or hematocrit. It is also important for your doctor to routinely check your hematocrit while on testosterone therapy to avoid increased risk of heart attack or stroke; too many red blood cells from the elevated testosterone levels could lead to an increased chance of heart attack or stroke.

If you're a man over forty, you should ask your doctor to draw your blood to test for testosterone levels. If you are dealing with less energy than you used to have, are having difficulty sleeping, or see negative changes in your physical appearance and strength, you may be suffering from diminished levels of testosterone. Testosterone replacement therapy could change your life, if it is found that your levels are not up to where they should be. You may even feel twenty-five again once you begin the therapy. But remember this—and this goes for men and women—the best results from HRT are achieved when a healthy, well-balanced diet and adequate exercise are practiced in conjunction with the therapy. If you don't exercise regularly, if you eat badly, or if you smoke, you will not see the results you desire.

Human Growth Hormone (HGH) for Anti-Aging

HGH is a peptide hormone that is produced and released by the pituitary gland, a pea-size structure at the base of the brain. This hormone gives way to childhood growth and also helps maintain tissues and organs throughout life. HGH medication is prescribed by physicians for use in slower-growing children and children genetically predisposed to dwarfism. The treatment generally begins for these children while they are in their preadolescent or adolescent years, at which point their epiphyseal plates, or "growth plates," in the long bones of the body have not yet calcified and stopped growing vertically.

As we age past our adolescent years, our natural production of growth hormone decreases. The levels then stabilize for us as adults until we reach our thirties or early forties, at which point a slow, steady decline in HGH production occurs.

This natural decrease in production and release of HGH with age has given way to an interest in the use of synthetic HGH to prevent or slow many age-related changes such as decreased muscle and bone mass, fine lines and wrinkles, hair loss, and lack of energy.

However grandiose HGH's fountain of youth—like tales and endorsements might be—there is very little evidence to suggest that HGH treatment can help healthy adults regain youth and vitality. Most physicians actually advise against using HGH to treat aging or age-related conditions due to the many possible side effects that go along with HGH therapy, some of which may be irreversible. Some of these side effects include acromegaly (the swelling and growth of certain soft tissues and organs), carpal tunnel syndrome, joint pain, fluid retention, and liver damage.

HGH is a very complex hormone and many of its functions are unknown at this time. However, athletes typically use HGH medication in an effort to speed up the recovery time or healing processes after extensive physical training, and bodybuilders use HGH medication to further their muscle growth. You don't have to look at research studies to notice acromegaly in certain people who abuse HGH. Just go to a top-level bodybuilding competition and you may find a few examples. With acromegaly, certain aesthetic traits are permanently altered. Examples of this include abnormally protruding forehead; growth of the nose, ears, hands, and feet; and distended gut due to growth of the internal organs.

The use of HGH in adults may be beneficial under certain circumstances. Adults who have true growth hormone deficiency, rather than just the expected decline in growth hormone due to aging, may benefit from prescription synthetic HGH. Growth hormone deficiency in adults is rare. For adults who have a growth hormone deficiency, injections of HGH can help improve their overall health by increasing bone density, muscle mass, and their exercise capacity, while also decreasing body fat. HGH is also used to treat adults with short bowel syndrome for growth and improved function of the bowels, as well as those who suffer from acquired immunodeficiency syndrome (AIDS) or human immunodeficiency virus (HIV) in order to help with AIDS-related muscle wasting.

CHAPTER 5

PLEASE DON'T SMOKE

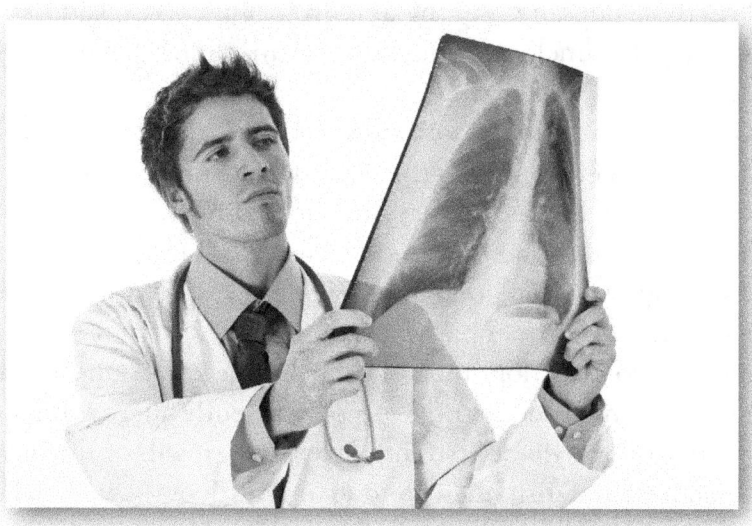

I CANNOT STRESS to you the gravity of smoking when it comes to your health. Furthermore, smoking ages you. If you currently smoke, get the proper help to quit immediately. If you don't smoke but at times think about it (particularly if you are a former smoker), erase such thoughts from your mind. If you're not a smoker but spend time with or live with a smoker, you are just as badly off as smoking yourself. Therefore, you will need to make the proper arrangements to somehow separate yourself from his or her smoking (if you cannot convince him or her to quit).

Smoking affects your health in countless ways, some of which you may not realize. Sure, it's associated with lung cancer—everyone knows that. But as dreadful as pulmonary carcinoma is, that's really just one of a large group of health conditions and diseases linked to smoking. The lungs are not by any means the only part of the body affected. Practically every aspect of the body is compromised in some form. Let's look at the organs of the body that suffer due to smoking.

LUNGS

This is the most obvious one, which everyone should be aware of by now. Physical effects in the lungs from smoking include scarred lung, destroyed lung tissue, and the paralysis or killing off of cilia within the airways.

SCARRED LUNG

Smoking causes inflammation in the small airways and tissues of the lungs. This causes the smoker to wheeze or feel short of breath. Continued inflammation will lead to the development and buildup of scar tissue, resulting in physical changes to the lungs and airways. This ultimately results in restricted breathing, making every breath more difficult. Over time, this lung irritation causes chronic cough.

EMPHYSEMA

Smoking destroys the tiny air sacs, known as alveoli, in the lungs, where oxygen is exchanged from the lungs into the bloodstream for distribution to all tissues of the body. These alveoli do not grow back or heal once they are destroyed. When enough alveoli are destroyed, emphysema develops, which is a serious condition that causes severe shortness of breath and may lead to death.[xxi]

RESPIRATORY INFECTIONS

Smoking also results in the paralysis or killing off of cilia in the airways. The cilia are tiny, hairlike fibers lining the airways that protect the airways and lungs from mucus and debris in the air, so they remain clear via a sweeping action elicited with each breath. Without the function of the cilia in the airways, the lungs are more prone to infection.

Immune System

Smoking leads to a weakened immune system. Cigarette smoke contains high levels of tar and other chemicals, which can cause the immune system to be less effective at fighting off infections. This is why smokers are more vulnerable to sickness, ranging anywhere from low-acuity conditions such as the cold or the flu, to more serious conditions such as autoimmune diseases, including rheumatoid arthritis and multiple sclerosis. Furthermore, with a weakened immune system, the body's ability to fight off cancer, regardless of the type or region of the body, is compromised.

Blood Changes

White blood cell (WBC) count is raised with smoking, which signifies increased stress on the body. WBCs are in the blood to help fight off infections, and the number of WBCs in the blood increases with stress. Increased WBC count typically signals that the body, or some part of the body, is injured. Over time, chronically high WBC counts can lead to heart attack, stroke, or even cancer.

Slowed Healing

Nicotine causes the blood vessels to constrict, resulting in decreased levels of nutrients supplied to tissues of the body. Consequently, healing is slowed by insufficient or less-than-optimal levels of nutrient supply to the wound area.

Damage to the Eyes

Smoking can threaten your eyesight. Nicotine restricts the production of a chemical known as rhodopsin, which is necessary for night vision. Also, smoking increases your risk of developing cataracts and macular degeneration, both of which can lead to blindness.

ERECTILE DYSFUNCTION

Due to nicotine's effect of vasoconstriction, there is less blood flow, including blood flow to the genital area. Without sufficient blood flow to the penis, the ability to get or keep an erection is decreased. Furthermore, certain toxins found in cigarette smoke can damage the genetic material in sperm, leading to infertility or genetic defects in the offspring.

DAMAGE TO DNA

All cells in the body contain genetic material, known as deoxyribonucleic acid (DNA), that acts as a blueprint for cell and tissue growth, development, and function. Smoking actually damages the DNA. When DNA is damaged, the genetic programming is altered, causing the cells affected to begin growing out of control, and quite possibly resulting in a cancer tumor. Our bodies are naturally designed to repair damage to the DNA, such as that undertaken by smoking; but over time, the body will succumb to the damages, as the repair system weakens from continuous damage from the toxins. At this point, the altered DNA that is not repaired properly may result in cancer. One-third of all cancer deaths are linked to tobacco use.

HEART DAMAGE

Blood pressure is raised by smoking, which increases the stress on the heart. Chronic increases in stress on the heart will cause this vital organ to weaken, making it less able to pump blood to all the organs and tissues of the body. Carbon monoxide from inhaled cigarette smoke also contributes to a lack of oxygen in the blood, placing an even tougher workload on the heart. This increases the risk of heart disease.

EFFECTS ON THE BRAIN

Nicotine has addictive properties that are similar to those of heroin.[xxii] Nicotine addiction is tough to conquer due to the effects it has on the brain. For smokers or users of other types of tobacco, the brain develops extra nicotine receptors to accommodate the large doses of nicotine from tobacco. When the brain stops getting the nicotine it's used to receiving, the result is nicotine withdrawal. Without smoking, the person trying to quit will feel anxious and irritable and have strong cravings for nicotine. Slowly, the cravings will fade with time as the unused nicotine receptors break down and degenerate, provided the ex-smoker does not give in and feed those needy nicotine receptors in the brain.

Weakened Bones

Certain chemicals in cigarette smoke disrupt the natural cycle of breakdown and renewal. The body is less able to form healthy new bone tissue and will break down existing bone tissue more rapidly. This leads to a loss of bone density, causing bones to become weak and brittle. The onset of osteopenia and osteoporosis is more likely in those who smoke. Smokers are at increased risk for fractures, and fractures that ensue are slower to heal than in nonsmokers.

Muscle Deterioration

In those who smoke, less blood flows to and from the muscle tissue. This results in a lack of nutrients and oxygen to the muscles, as well as a decrease in toxin removal and waste removal from the muscles. This results in less ability to build or maintain muscle tissue.

Skin Aging

Smoking leads to dryness and loss of elasticity in the skin, resulting in wrinkles and stretch marks. The skin tone becomes dull and grayish in smokers. It is not uncommon for people in their thirties who smoke to show signs of aging in the skin that are similar to forty- or fifty-somethings, due to the destructive effects of smoking. When you smoke, your blood vessels immediately become thinner and spasm, constricting blood flow, reducing circulation and oxygen in the blood. If you reduce circulation, you reduce the delivery of nutrients and oxygen to your skin. Without the proper nutrients and oxygen, less essential nutrition is given to the collagen fibers, elastin fibers, and all supporting tissues of the dermis. As these structures are compromised, the skin will lose strength and elasticity. With this loss of robustness in the skin, wrinkles form, as the underlying fibers that previously held the skin tight and firm have been starved of the proper nutrients and oxygen. This is one of the many irreversible effects of smoking, and the more you smoke, the more damage that is done.

The Dangers of Nicotine

As awful as cigarette smoking is, other forms of tobacco use are no less detrimental. Take smokeless chew, for example. Tobacco chew is potentially an even higher threat than smoking for a couple of reasons. For one, nicotine is transferred very quickly through direct contact with the gums, significantly increasing the chance of cancer in the gums or throat, more so than cigarette smoking. Second, chew gives a person more of a sensation of alertness, compared to smoking, making it very addictive. This sense of alertness is actually increased blood pressure, due to the vasoconstriction of the blood vessels.

Nicotine is most dangerous on a chemical level, as it reduces the amount of antioxidants such as vitamins and minerals within the blood that are usually present to ward off free radicals in the blood and tissues. This is more significant in smoking than with the use of tobacco in other forms, as the by-products of cigarette smoke include certain carcinogenic chemicals and free radicals.

Many people who smoke feel that they are more mentally alert and focused after smoking. This, in addition to nicotine's intensely addictive properties, gives smokers a way to rationalize continuing this harmful habit. To actually believe tobacco improves performance or enhances alertness is to ignore the preponderance of evidence that it harms the body. Within seconds after the puff of a cigarette or the insertion of chew into the mouth, unfavorable chemical changes begin to take place in the bloodstream and in the entire body.

If you are a smoker, you should contact your doctor right away and ask him or her to help you establish a smoking-cessation plan. Certain prescription medications are available, as well as over-the-counter nicotine patches and gums. In addition, a therapist, psychologist, or psychiatrist may also be of great benefit in kicking the habit. Many studies also conclude that hypnotherapy is a great tool for quitting smoking.

Surrounding yourself with nonsmokers and spending less time with friends and family members who smoke may be very helpful. There may be countless changes in your lifestyle that need to take place in order for you to rid yourself of the smoking habit, but it is truly worth it. Smoking cessation is by no means easy for most people, but it can certainly be achieved, no matter how long you have smoked. As Mark Twain once said, "It's easy to quit smoking: I've done it a hundred times." If you simply decide to quit cold turkey, without the use of medications, modalities, or therapy, your chances of success are not in your favor. You need a plan—one that helps lower your cravings for cigarette smoking, helps you through tough times when you're craving a drag, and allows you to realize the positive aspects of no longer having to smoke to enjoy life.

CHAPTER 6

KEEP A VIBRANT, YOUTHFUL OUTLOOK

YOUR ATTITUDE MAKES all the difference. For instance, remember Jeanne Calment, the French lady who lived to the ripe age of 122? If you study her life and the people who knew her, you will find that by most accounts, she did not stress the small things. She would not worry about things, because she realized that worrying accomplished nothing. She also rode a bike up until the age of one hundred, and walked all over her town to thank everyone who congratulated her on her hundredth birthday that year.

The late Mrs. Calment's positive attitude is a good example of how you should strive to view your life. Stressing the small things in your life will not usually help matters. Only actions may help but not worrying. If you find yourself under lots of mental or emotional stress at your workplace, aside from quitting your job and moving on to a less demanding one, you might consider various stress-relieving techniques or activities. You should take vacations. You should make it part of your weekly, monthly, and yearly regimens to take time for yourself by doing the things you enjoy. If traveling makes you happy, do it more. If going to the park to feed the pigeons is peaceful to you, go there and do that at least once a week for a couple hours. Whatever you can do to relax and enjoy life's pleasures, make that a bigger part of your life. Soon, you will find yourself happier and full of energy, having a better mental attitude, and maybe even feeling younger.

A positive mental attitude is the path to a forever-youthful life. Maintaining a positive outlook on life impacts your perception of youth. If you want to delay the process of aging, you must feel, think, and act young in hopes that your body will take action based on what the mind thinks. In other words, you must want to stay young. Just as Rhonda Byrne mentions in her very famous *New York Times* best seller, *The Secret*, your mind is the key to having what you want in life.[xxiii] So, if you desire to feel young again, you must focus on that idea, make the proper adjustments in your life to achieve your idea of feeling more youthful and full of energy, and your path will be laid out for the reality of feeling twenty-five again.

Most people don't believe the power of their own minds. However, it directly affects what their actions will be. That is the idea behind Byrne's *The Secret* as well as teachings of many of the world's best-known philosophers. What your mind portrays is reflected on the outside, so you act on whatever is in your mind. If you feel depressed or lethargic, chances are that you will continue on this downward spiral of lethargy, unless something causes your mind to change and stop the negative feelings. So, remember to think positively more often, do more things that make you happy and put your mind at ease, and avoid people or situations that put you in a negative state of mind as much as possible.

Focus on Keeping a Healthy Attitude at All Times

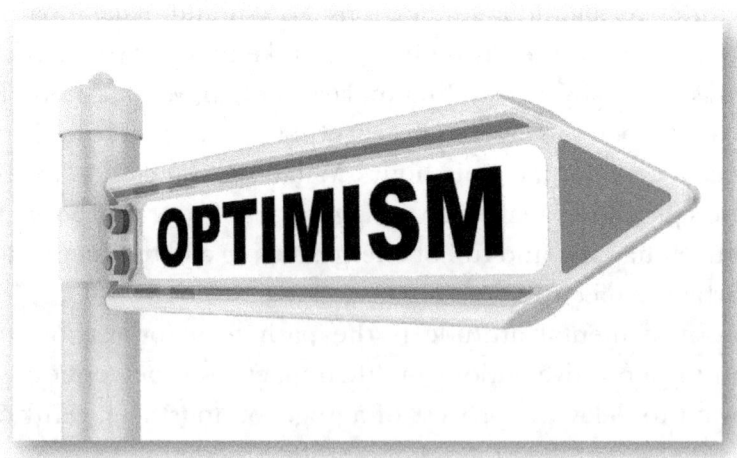

Maintaining a state of positive thinking, even when things don't seem to be going your way, may be quite challenging. You will need practice, but you can change the way you handle the mental and emotional burdens that so commonly bring you down. There are a few methods for placing yourself in an environment that encourages a positive outlook.

SURROUND YOURSELF WITH HAPPIER PEOPLE

Do your friends, family, or colleagues play a role in making you think negatively? Do any of your contacts have only negative things to say about anything and everything? Are there people you're around daily or weekly who seem to never have anything good to say about practically anything because they focus so much on the negatives all the time? Are you surrounded by pessimists? Or even worse, are you stuck with people who tend to bully and demean you?

Constant association with negative thinkers and pessimists can be daunting to anybody but even more so for someone who is attempting to be just the opposite. These people will drain you of energy and emotionally exhaust you with their constant bullying and manipulation.

Your general well-being is easily influenced by those around you. If you can keep this in mind, you will have a greater understanding of the quality of your social interactions and how they affect you. Remember also that everything you say or do affects others around you. Simply by sharing space with others who are negative out in public, in a room, out on the sidewalk, in the office, wherever—if you are around them for even just a few minutes, you will likely pick up on their energy, how they feel, and more, without meaning to do so. Sadness, anger, irritability, and worry are contagious. That said, so are happiness, joy, and positive thinking.

By surrounding yourself with people who think positively and are generally happy, you cancel out much of the negativity that may be around you, and in doing so, you encourage more nurturing and supportive energy for yourself. Such an atmosphere of positive people surrounding you more often will allow for better understanding, love, and respect for you and for your family, friends, and colleagues.

Just remember to select your friends and close acquaintances carefully, as they create the environment you live in, be it a nurturing and positive one, or a draining and negative one. It is a good idea to give everyone the opportunity to be a friend, but spend your time only with those who will not bring you down due to their constant negativity or lack of concern for your thoughts, goals, and dreams.

WORK ON YOUR SELF-ESTEEM

Self-esteem is basically how you feel about yourself, what you think you deserve in life, and how your rate yourself in relation to others. With a healthy self-esteem, you hold a sense of high self-worth, you believe that you are deserving of love and happiness, and you have a high level of confidence in accomplishing your goals and other tasks in life. Having a high level of self-esteem is closely related to the topic just discussed— you will need to refrain from mingling with the negative thinkers around you and instead have more dealings with those who are uplifting and caring for you and your goals. If you do not separate from those who are exhausting you mentally and emotionally, you will end up with low self-esteem and self-worth. Having low self-esteem can be detrimental to your mental and physical health. When you have feelings of low self-esteem that are compounded by negative emotions such as anxiety, depression, and emotional stress, you significantly increase the risk of heart disease.[xxiv]

Low self-esteem or persistent negative thoughts and feelings will inadvertently cause the body to release certain stress hormones that will actually weaken the immune system and increase inflammation. This results in an increased likelihood of contracting an illness. Another problem with this reaction is the resultant tearing down of healthy protein tissues and an increase in body-fat storage. And perhaps more detrimental than anything else is the strong correlation between low self-esteem and heart disease, increased LDL (bad cholesterol), lowered HDL (good cholesterol), and raised triglycerides.

If you have low self-esteem, your level of stress is increased as a result, which may lead you into unhealthy behaviors such as smoking and alcohol abuse. This is evidenced in a rather illuminating study by Andrew Steptoe and colleagues at University College London, published in a 1998 edition of the *British Journal of Health Psychology*: "Stress, Hassles and Variations in Alcohol Consumption, Food Choice and Physical Exercise: A Diary Study."[xxv] Obviously, diminished self-esteem and unhealthy behaviors such as smoking and excessive drinking are an unhealthy combination, sure to affect your social behavior. In such a scenario, you may find you have diminished incentive to properly care for yourself with diet, exercise, and other aspects needed to maintain a healthier you.

Conversely, having a healthy level of self-esteem can improve your mental and physical health. If you want to enjoy life the way life is meant to be appreciated and embraced, you will need a more positive outlook on things, including your view of yourself.

Healthy self-esteem will allow you to enjoy positive emotions such as gratitude, joy, pleasure, and relaxation. These positive emotions actually help protect your body from stress and its associated side effects—such positivity is conducive to good mental and physical health. Happiness, joyfulness, and a positive outlook on life may offer longevity and prosperity.

Do the Things That Excite You

There is not much use in living on this earth if you don't allow yourself to go out and engage in the activities that you enjoy. This is equally true for things that may excite you, yet possibly scare you a little bit. For instance, you may have always wanted to go bungee jumping. However, after years and years of considering going out and giving it a try, you still haven't gone for it. My advice to you is to make a list of the activities you enjoy doing that you've done before; another list of things that you've always wanted to do but have not yet done; and another list of things you're interested in doing that nevertheless scare you.

Perform this exercise, and then after jotting down all you can think of, rank the ones you are most interested in doing within each individual category by placing a number beside each item. Highlight the top three items from each category.

- Things I enjoy doing that I've done before or do regularly:

- Things I want to try for the first time that do not scare me:

- Things I want to try for the first time that scare me:

Your top three picks from each category are the activities you should do right away. Make a goal to accomplish all three from the first column within the next thirty days. As for the second and third columns, give yourself one year to complete the top three from each of these lists. Whether it's a simple road trip that covers areas you've never driven or a month-long tour of Europe, do your best to make this happen within the next 365 days. You may not see this as an exercise that deals with anti-aging, but indeed, it is. Without joy and excitement in your life, you age psychologically, socially, and spiritually. The intangible aspects of your health are being deprived of positive stimuli, which may result in a cascade of events that lead to negativity and can ultimately affect physical health. Life is short, and you only live once.

There are no guarantees in life either. So fill your life with as much joy and splendor as you can.

ENJOY MORE SEX

It's true—sex can help you stay young. In an interview reported in BBC News online, neuropsychologist David Weeks explained that couples who have sex at least three times a week look more than ten years younger than the average adult who makes love twice a week, according to his findings from a ten-year study of the subject. Weeks explained that there are chemical factors as well as emotional and physical ones that contribute to the health benefits. He explained that sexual intercourse is the most intense kind of pleasure, triggering the release of certain chemicals in the body, such as human growth hormone, which have an effect on anti-aging and health, among other healthful chemicals.[xxvi]

According to Weeks, regular, loving sex came second to physical and mental activity as the factors most important to retaining youth. In the study, he and his colleagues discovered that people can benefit from working and socializing with younger and older people and from having younger partners. The study also concluded that people who look younger are more altruistic, confident, and have more intellectual activity.

Weeks did, however, point out that it is loving intercourse with a regular partner, and not promiscuous sexual activity, that brings about the most benefit. "Casual sex would bring a lot of the detrimental things to staying youthful such as anxiety and the absence of security. Both those things are associated with a loss of youth," stated Weeks. The findings from Weeks's research are described in detail in a book that he coauthored, *Superyoung: The Proven Way to Stay Young Forever.*[xxvii]

TAKE MORE VACATIONS

If you're not one to leave your town that often, and you usually elect not to venture out and explore other parts of the country, continent, or world, you are not *truly* living. One of my all-time favorite books—*The 4-Hour*

Workweek: Escape 9–5, Live Anywhere, and Join the New Rich by Timothy Ferriss—explains this concept so well. As both a raving fan of his *New York Times* best-seller book and his iTunes top-rated business podcasts, I highly recommend following him on the various social media networks and utilizing his material. Much of what Ferriss preaches is the notion of rearranging one's life in such a way as to allow for extended vacations regularly, as opposed to working all the time, rarely/if ever taking a vacation, and waiting until retirement to travel. Ferriss refers to these regularly practiced, extended vacations as "mini-retirements."[xxviii]

Traveling to new places and immersing yourself in other cultures can be of so much benefit in several parameters. It is invigorating, stress relieving, encourages activity, and is great for your mental, physical, and spiritual health and well-being.

Taking a break from your typical daily routine may help to relieve your stress simply by providing a change of scenery. The excitement of getting ready for a trip can be a euphoric experience, and just the anticipation alone can take your mind off the petty problems that may at times seem larger than life to you. Getting away from your typical, mundane experience will allow you to take a step back and discern what you actually find important in your life.

Immersing yourself in a new location or culture will help you realize a new perspective on life. Through meeting different people with fresh experiences and ideas, showing you varying takes on life, you can immensely expand your mind. Each new setting you immerse yourself in will provide anonymity that gives you the luxury of freeing yourself to enjoy life.

Meeting new people will give you the opportunity to learn the different methods people use to accomplish the same goals, unveiling new ideas that you may have previously never thought of. A different social setting from what you're used to will help you appreciate the uniqueness of yourself and all you have to offer to the world.

Seeing new places and enjoying different cultures keep you young and fueled with energy. Such experiences can give you clarity and a broader mind and may allow you to gain much new knowledge of the world.

LAUGH MORE

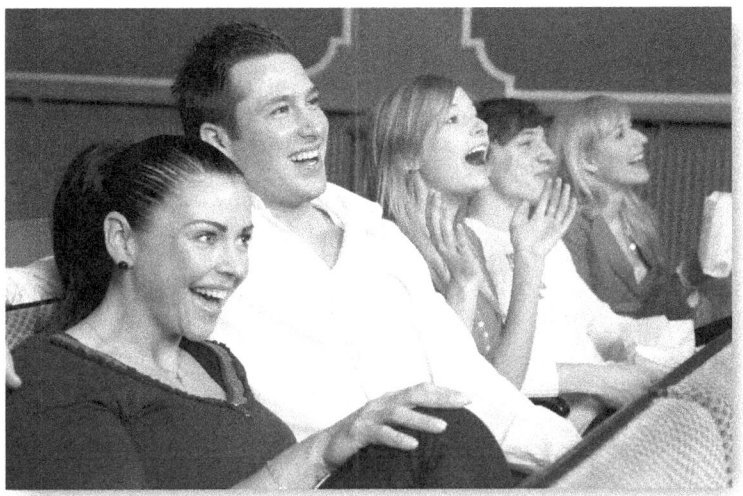

The healing power of laughter is real. You can't focus too heavily on all of the negative things going on in your life when you're laughing about something. Laughter is a powerful antidote to stress, pain, and conflict. There's nothing like a good laugh for bringing your mind and body back into balance. Humor helps relieve your mind of emotional and psychological burdens, connects you to others, and keeps you grounded and alert.

In a study in which formal humor and creative play was incorporated into a collaborative work environment, notable improvement in the work outcome was observed. The study effectively demonstrated that on-the-job playfulness improves communication, creativity, problem solving, and team building, thereby increasing productivity and satisfaction.[xxix]

There are also studies demonstrating that laughter may contribute to a lower prevalence of cardiovascular diseases. An article published in the *Journal of Epidemiology* in 2016 reported such a correlation. This was a cross-sectional study comprised of 20,934 individuals (10,206 men and 10,728 women) aged sixty-five years or older, who participated in the Japan Gerontological Evaluation Study in 2013. In the mail-in survey, participants provided information on daily frequency of laughter as well as body mass index, demographic and lifestyle factors, and diagnoses of cardiovascular disease, hyperlipidemia, hypertension, and depression. Even after adjustment for hyperlipidemia, hypertension, depression, body mass index, and other risk factors, the prevalence of heart diseases among those who never or almost never laughed was over 20 percent higher than those who reported laughing every day.[xxx]

Possessing the ability to laugh easily and frequently is a tremendous resource for overcoming your problems, enhancing your relationships, and facilitating improvement in physical and emotional well-being. Having a good, healthy sense of humor helps you maintain a positive, optimistic outlook through difficult situations, disappointments, losses, and failures.

Conclusion

By now, you should recognize that anti-aging and healthy living are so intertwined that when you are in discussion about one, in most respects, you are essentially talking about the other. From diet and nutrition to exercise and fitness, to having a healthy and positive attitude, you must choose to take excellent care of yourself on the outside as well as from within in order to look and feel younger. There is really no age-defying treatment out there that, in the long term, will substitute for living a healthy lifestyle. Sure, by all means, have cosmetic procedures to turn back the clock for aesthetic purposes if it helps with your self-esteem and helps you to feel younger and better looking, but that does not fix anything beyond the outer layer. If you want to truly stay as young as you can, you must take care of your body from within. Always remember that free radicals damage your body's cells and therefore will age you. You should seek to fight them off with a lifestyle that guards against these damaging chemicals floating around in the body and out in the air we breathe every day.

Aging is not just about how old you are but also how old you *feel*. There are studies demonstrating that an optimistic outlook on life results in both a longer life and more life to the years. After all, what is the use in living if you are not enjoying the time spent in your life? Don't you think life is meant to be enjoyed? Well, you won't enjoy nearly as many years living a life that tears your body and soul down with stress, free radicals, and negativity. Remember this little tip the next time you go for a cheeseburger at a fast-food joint. Also, keep it in mind when you are in a stressful situation that consumes you, whether it be with time, energy, worry, or all of the above.

Also, please keep in mind that you need to see the humor in life. There are studies to back up the much-believed idea that people with a greater sense of humor live longer. Furthermore, we can assume that seeing the humor in life results in a greater enjoyment of life. So, try to see the funny side of things. Don't dwell on problems, losses, and fears so much. Try to compartmentalize such negative thoughts, feelings, and emotions and focus your attention on things that make you laugh. The healing power of laughter is real. Redirecting your attention to something you find to be funny is a quick solution to being down in the dumps.

You have only so many years on this earth, and you only live once. Maximize it by taking care of yourself, enjoying the time you have here, and living a life that's truly worth living.

About the Author

Dr. Courtney Alan Mote, also referred to as Corey Mote, is a chiropractic physician, professional natural bodybuilder, fitness model, spokesperson, and columnist for many fitness magazines and medical/healthcare journals in North America and abroad. He has been the featured subject of many fitness magazines internationally. He is the owner and operator of a multidisciplinary medical practice north of Atlanta, Georgia. For more information on Dr. Mote, please visit his website at www.coreymote.com.

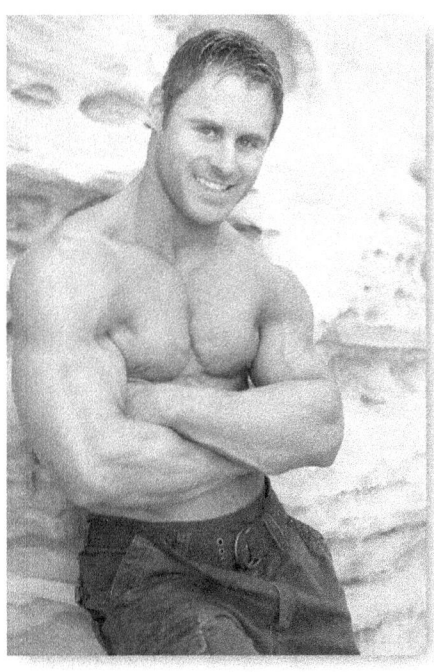

Endnotes

Chapter One

i.   Nicholas Perricone, *The Wrinkle Cure: Unlock the Power of Cosmeceuticals for Supple, Youthful Skin* (New York: Rodale Books, 2005). Read this book at http://www.amazon.com/The-Wrinkle-Cure-Cosmeceuticals-Youthful/dp/0446617172.

ii.   See http://news.yahoo.com/health-benefits-greek-yogurt-120000389.html.

iii.   Toby Amidor, *The Greek Yogurt Kitchen: More Than 130 Delicious, Healthy Recipes for Every Meal of the Day* (New York: Grand Central Publishing, 2014). Read this book at http://www.amazon.com/The-Greek-Yogurt-Kitchen-Delicious/dp/1455551201.

iv.   L. Heilbronn and E. Ravussin, "Calorie Restriction and Aging: Review of the Literature and Implications for Studies in Humans," *American Journal of Clinical Nutrition 78, no. 3 (2003): 361–369.*

v.   Montash University, "Killer Carbs: Scientist Finds Key to Overeating as We Age," *Science Daily.* Retrieved February 10, 2016 (www.sciencedaily.com/releases/2008/08/080821110113.htm).

vi.   Jacqueline Chan et al., "Water, Other Fluids, and Fatal Coronary Heart Disease: The Adventist Health Study," *American Journal of Epidemiology* 155, no. 3 (2002): 827–833.

vii.   Brenda Davy, "Clinical Trial Confirms Effectiveness of Simple Appetite Control Method," paper presented at the American Chemical Society National Meeting, Boston, Massachusetts,

August 23, 2010. (http://www.acs.org/content/acs/en/pressroom/ newsreleases/2010/august/clinical-trial-confirms-effectiveness-of-simple-appetite-control-method.html).

viii. Peter Bennett and Stephen Barrie, *7-Day Detox Miracle: Revitalize Your Mind and Body with This Safe and Effective Life-Enhancing Program* (New York: Three Rivers Press, 2001). Read this book at http://www.amazon.com/gp/product/B004QWZHEC/ ref=dp-kindle-redirect?ie=UTF8&btkr=1.

Chapter Two

ix. F. B. Schuch et al., "Exercise as a Treatment for Depression: A Meta-Analysis Adjusting for Publication Bias," *Journal of Psychiatric Research* 77 (2016): 42–51.

x. M. Kleinstäuber et al., "Pharmacological Interventions for Somatoform Disorders in Adults," *Cochrane Database System Review* 11 (2014): CD010628.

xi. National Sleep Foundation, "Exercise and Sleep." Retrieved January 16, 2016
(https://sleepfoundation.org/sleep-topics/exercise-and-sleep).

xii. EurekAlert, "Brief Exercise Reduces Impact of Stress on Cell Aging, UCSF Study shows." Retrieved January 23, 2016
(http://www.eurekalert.org/pub_releases/2010-05/uoc-- ber052510.php).

xiii. Marie-Noel Vercambre et al., "Physical Activity and Cognition in Women with Vascular Conditions," *Archives of Internal Medicine* 171, no. 14 (2011): 1244–1250.

xiv. J. L. Talanian et al., "Two Weeks of High-Intensity Aerobic Interval Training Increases the Capacity for Fat Oxidation during Exercise in Women," *Journal of Applied Physiology* 102, no. 4 (2007): 1439–1447.

Chapter Three

xv. Lisa Drayer, "The Top 10 Superfoods for Gorgeous Skin and Hair," *Fitness*. Retrieved February 16, 2016 (http://www.fitnessmagazine.com/recipes/healthy-eating/superfoods/top-10-superfoods-for-skin-and-hair/).

xvi. C. Adebamowo et al., "Milk Consumption and Acne in Teenaged Boys," *Journal of the American Academy of Dermatology* 58, no. 5 (2008): 787–793.

xvii. Denise Mann, "Are We Pushing the Antiaging Envelope?" *WebMD*. Retrieved January 25, 2016 (http://www.webmd.com/beauty/botox/are-we-pushing-antiaging-envelope).

xviii. R. Morgan Griffin, "What's the Best Sunscreen?" *WebMD*. Retrieved January 12, 2016 (http://www.webmd.com/beauty/sun/whats-best-sunscreen).

Chapter Four

xix. Mayo Clinic, "Testosterone Therapy: Potential Benefits and Risks as You Age." Retrieved April 1, 2015. (http://www.mayoclinic.org/healthy-lifestyle/sexual-health/in-depth/testosterone-therapy/art-20045728).

xx. F. Saad et al., "A Dose-Response Study of Testosterone on Sexual Dysfunction and Features of the Metabolic Syndrome Using

Testosterone Gel and Parenteral Testosterone Undecanoate," *Journal of Andrology* 29, no. 1 (2008): 102–105.

Chapter Five

xxi.   "Emphysema In-Depth Report," *The New York Times*. Retrieved February 2, 2016 (http://www.nytimes.com/health/guides/disease/emphysema/print.html).

xxii. F. E. Pontieri et al., "Effects of Nicotine on the Nucleus Accumbens and Similarity to Those of Addictive Drugs," *Nature* 382, no. 6588 (1996): 255–257.

Chapter Six

xxiii. Rhonda Byrne, *The Secret* (New York: Atria Books, 2006). Read this book at http://www.amazon.com/gp/product/B002M5E2DW/ref=dp-kindle-redirect?ie=UTF8&btkr=1.

xxiv. A. O'Neil et al., "Depression Is a Risk Factor for Incident Coronary Heart Disease in Women: An 18-Year Longitudinal Study," *Journal of Affective Disorders* 196 (2016): 117–124.

xxv.   A. Steptoe, Z. Lipsey, and J. Wardle, "Stress, Hassles and Variations in Alcohol Consumption, Food Choice and Physical Exercise: A Diary Study," *British Journal of Health Psychology* 3 (1998): 51–63.

xxvi. "Sex Keeps You Young," *BBC News*. Retrieved March 10, 1999. (http://news.bbc.co.uk/2/hi/health/294119.stm).

xxvii. Jamie James and David Weeks, *Superyoung: The Proven Way to Stay Young Forever* (London: Hodder, 1999). Read this book at http://www.amazon.co.uk/The-Superyoung-proven-young-forever-x/dp/0340682345.

xxviii. Timothy Ferriss, *The 4-Hour Workweek: Escape 9–5, Live Anywhere, and Join the New Rich* (New York: Crown, 2007). Read this book at http://www.amazon.com/dp/B002WE46UW/ref=r_soa_w_d.

xxix. R. Burchiel and C. King, "Incorporating Fun into the Business of Serious Work: The Use of Humor in Group Process," *Seminars in Perioperative Nursing* 8, no. 2 (1999): 60–70.

xxx. K. Hayashi et al., "Laughter Is the Best Medicine? A Cross-Sectional Study of Cardiovascular Disease among Older Japanese Adults," *Journal of Epidemiology* (2016).

www.ingramcontent.com/pod-product-compliance
Lightning Source LLC
Chambersburg PA
CBHW07221328056
45788CB00002B/1006